Black Psychiatrists and American Psychiatry

Black Psychiatrists and American Psychiatry

Edited by
JEANNE SPURLOCK, M.D.

Foreword by John Hope Franklin

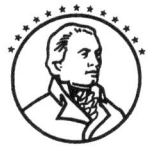

Published by the American Psychiatric Association
WASHINGTON, DC

Note: The authors have worked to ensure that all information in this book concerning drug dosages, schedules, and routes of administration is accurate as of the time of publication and consistent with standards set by the U.S. Food and Drug Administration and the general medical community. As medical research and practice advance, however, therapeutic standards may change. For this reason and because human and mechanical errors sometimes occur, we recommend that readers follow the advice of a physician who is directly involved in their care or the care of a member of their family.

The findings, opinions, and conclusions of this publication do not necessarily represent the views of the officers, trustees, or all members of the American Psychiatric Association. The views expressed are those of the authors of the individual chapters.

Copyright © 1999 American Psychiatric Association

ALL RIGHTS RESERVED

First Edition
02 01 00 99 4 3 2

American Psychiatric Association
1400 K Street, N.W.
Washington, DC 20005
www.psych.org

Library of Congress Cataloging-in-Publication Data
Black psychiatrists and American psychiatry / edited by Jeanne
  Spurlock. Foreword by John Hope Franklin.—1st ed.
      p.   cm.
  Includes bibliographical references and index.
  ISBN 0-89042-411-X
  1. Afro-American psychiatrists—Biography. 2. Afro-American
psychiatrists—History.   I. Spurlock, Jeanne.   II. Franklin, John Hope.
  [DNLM: 1. Psychiatry—United States. 2. Psychiatry personal
narratives. 3. Blacks—United States. WM 21B627 1999]
RC438.5.B63   1999
616.89′008996′073—dc21
DNLM/DLC
for Library of Congress   98-36902
                                                                     CIP

British Library Cataloguing in Publication Data
A CIP record is available from the British Library.

Contents

Contributors   *vii*
Foreword, John Hope Franklin, Ph.D.   *xi*
Preface, Jeanne Spurlock, M.D.   *xv*

Part I: Historical Reviews

1. Early and Contemporary Pioneers   3
   Jeanne Spurlock, M.D.
2. Development of a Department of Psychiatry in a General Hospital   25
   Elizabeth B. Davis, M.D.
3. Community Psychiatry and Work in the Public Sector, 1962–1980   47
   June Jackson Christmas, M.D.
4. Development of the Department of Psychiatry at Meharry Medical College   67
   Lloyd C. Elam, M.D.
5. Participant Observer: The Experiences of a Black Transcultural Psychiatrist   77
   Victor R. Adebimpe, M.D.
6. Black Americans in Military Psychiatry   95
   Clotilde Dent Bowen, M.D., F.A.P.M., (L.)APA, Col. U.S. Army (Ret.)
   James L. Collins Sr., M.D., F.A.P.A., Col. U.S. Army (Ret.)

Part II: Surveys

7. Black Psychiatrists and Academia   109
   Irma J. Bland, M.D.
   Bruce L. Ballard, M.D.
8. Child and Adolescent Psychiatrists   129
   Donna M. Norris, M.D.
   Joshua W. Calhoun, M.D.
   Ruth L. Fuller, M.D.
   Harry H. Wright, M.D., M.B.A.

9. Black Psychiatric Researchers — 141
   F.M. Baker, M.D., M.P.H.
   Tana A. Grady-Weliky, M.D.

10. Forensic Psychiatry — 153
    Ledro R. Justice, M.D.

11. Black Psychoanalysts — 163
    Ruth L. Fuller, M.D.
    Jeanne Spurlock, M.D.
    Hugh F. Butts, M.D.
    Henry E. Edwards, M.D.

Part III: Personal Reminiscences

12. Reflections of a Commissioner of Mental Health and a Head of a Department of Psychiatry — 179
    Mildred Mitchell-Bateman, M.D.

13. Reflections on the Career of a Black Psychiatrist in the Veterans Administration — 187
    James E. Baker, M.D.

Part IV: Current Mental Health Issues Affecting Black Americans

14. Current Mental Health Issues Affecting Black Americans — 205
    Billy E. Jones, M.D., M.S.

Index — 217

Contributors

Victor R. Adebimpe, M.D.
Medical Director, Adult Psychiatry, Mercy Psychiatric Institute,
  Pittsburgh, Pennsylvania

F. M. Baker, M.D., M.P.H.
Professor, Department of Psychiatry, John A. Burns School of Medicine,
  University of Hawaii at Manoa Hawaii State Hospital, Kaneohe, Hawaii

James E. Baker, M.D.
Associate Chief, Treatment Services, Veterans Administration (Ret.),
  Williamsburg, Virginia

Bruce L. Ballard, M.D.
Associate Dean, Cornell University Medical College, New York, New York

Irma J. Bland, M.D.
Associate Professor of Psychiatry, Louisiana State University College of
  Medicine; Regional Medical Director, Office of Mental Health, New
  Orleans, Louisiana

Clotilde Dent Bowen, M.D., F.A.P.M., (L.)APA
Colonel, United States Army (Ret.); Staff Psychiatrist, Veterans
  Administration Hospital, Colorado Springs, Colorado (Ret.)

Hugh F. Butts, M.D.
Adjunct Professor, Psychiatry, New York College of Podiatric Medicine;
  Psychiatric Consultant, Columbia Law School, New York, New York

Joshua W. Calhoun, M.D.
Chair, Division of Child and Adolescent Psychiatry, St. John's Mercy
  Medical Center, St. Louis, Missouri

June Jackson Christmas, M.D.
Clinical Professor of Psychiatry, Columbia University of Physicians
  and Surgeons; Executive Director, Urban Issues Group, New York,
  New York

Contributors

James L. Collins Sr., M.D., F.A.P.A.
Colonel, United States Army (Ret.); Clinical Director, Crownsville Hospital Center, Crownsville, Maryland

Elizabeth B. Davis, M.D.
Professor Emeritus, Psychiatry, Columbia University, College of Physicians and Surgeons, New York, New York

Henry E. Edwards, M.D.
Mental Health Consultant, District of Columbia Department of Corrections; Consultant, St. Elizabeths Hospital and Walter Reed Hospital Departments of Psychiatry, Washington, DC

Lloyd C. Elam, M.D.
Professor in Psychiatry; Former President; Dean; Chairperson, Department of Psychiatry, Meharry Medical College, Nashville, Tennessee

John Hope Franklin, Ph.D.
James B. Duke Professor Emeritus, Department of History, Duke University, Durham, North Carolina

Ruth L. Fuller, M.D.
Associate Professor of Psychiatry, University of Colorado, Health Sciences Center, Denver, Colorado

Tana A. Grady-Weliky, M.D.
Associate Dean for Undergraduate Medical Education, University of Rochester School of Medicine, Rochester, New York

Billy E. Jones, M.D., M.S.
Former Commissioner, New York City Department of Mental Health, Mental Retardation and Alcoholism Services; Former President, New York City Health and Hospitals Corporation; Senior Vice President and Medical Director, Public Sector, Magellan Health Services, New York, New York

Ledro R. Justice, M.D.
Medical Director, Jefferson School, Jefferson, Maryland; Assistant Professor, Psychiatry and Pediatrics, George Washington University School of Medicine, Washington, DC

Mildred Mitchell-Bateman, M.D.
Professor, Psychiatry, Marshall University School of Medicine; Associate

Clinical Director, Huntington State Hospital, Huntington, West Virginia

Donna M. Norris, M.D.
Private Practice, Wellesley, Massachusetts, Instructor, Psychiatry, Harvard University School of Medicine, Boston, Massachusetts

Jeanne Spurlock, M.D.
Clinical Professor of Psychiatry, George Washington School of Medicine and Health Sciences and Howard University College of Medicine, Washington, DC

Harry H. Wright, M.D., M.B.A.
Professor of Psychiatry, University of South Carolina School of Medicine, Columbia, South Carolina

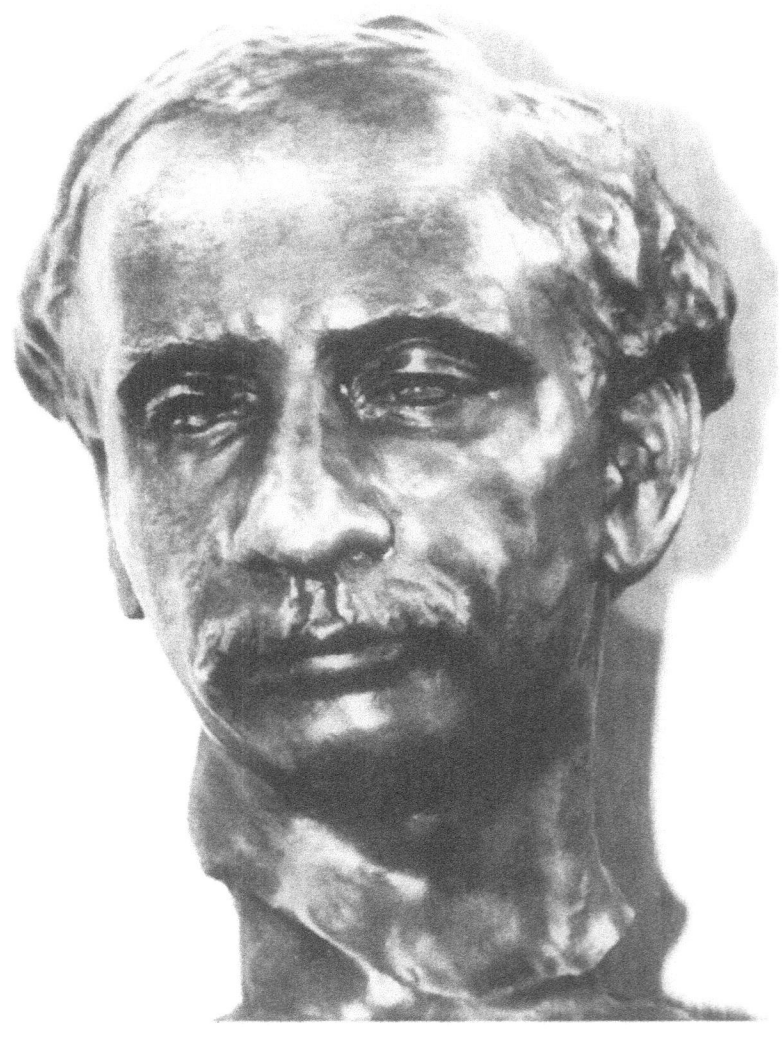

Bust of Dr. Solomon Carter Fuller, located in the lobby of the Dr. Solomon Carter Fuller Mental Health Center in Boston, Massachusetts

—Photo by Eugene Bussey, Roxbury, MA

Foreword

Those who work in the field of history can readily appreciate the importance of delineating as complete a picture as possible as one seeks to reconstruct the past. Those who work in the field of black American history have the additional burden of making certain that the distortions and misrepresentations of earlier writers in the field do not influence the necessary effort to provide a quite different version of what happened in the past. The special problems that black Americans have faced in finding a place to live in neighborhoods where no other members of their race lived; the difficulties they have confronted in seeking employment in a hostile workplace; and their confusing and frustrating attempts to find a place of worship, which brought stares and sneers from their would-be fellow communicants, indicate a few of the challenges that black Americans have experienced while trying to find their niche in the larger American community.

The situation is infinitely more difficult in areas where the objective is presumably to discover the truth without the distractions of preconceptions born of prejudice. The remarkable fact is that in some fields of inquiry, where scientific truth should be the hallmark of judging persons or, indeed, discoveries, some of the most rigid and inhospitable attitudes toward certain human beings working in the same field have been manifested. It is as if the scientist, looking up from the microscope or mathematical equation, had seen a black American would-be colleague and had reacted as if the entire scientific inquiry had been spoiled by the intrusion. It is enormously important that the experiences of persons seeking to enter new fields be recorded not only to provide an instrument by which change is measured but also to indicate some guidelines for future aspirants as they seek to further their own careers in a given vocation.

Unhappily, experiences such as these can be found in virtually every area of human endeavor in the United States. The long battle that black Americans had to wage merely to gain admission to numerous colleges and universities—not all in the South, incidentally—indicate that resistance is strong in the very places where judgments should be made on considerations other than the color of one's skin. The situation has been particularly perplexing in graduate and professional schools, where the last vestiges of prejudice based on race and gender should have disappeared long ago. Perhaps the most remarkable thing of all is that black Americans were barred from some of the very best graduate and professional schools for the flimsiest, most unscientific reasons imaginable. If by chance they were successful in securing their training, then the scientific and professional societies spurned their quest for membership, thus depriving them further of an opportunity to benefit from collegial association.

Black psychiatrists have had more than their share of experiences of discrimination, loss of opportunity for growth through professional association, and deprivation of the opportunity for experimentation and study so necessary for anyone attempting to remain part of a burgeoning field. Yet the history of black American psychiatrists, especially as delineated in this work, is the history of a relatively small group of well-trained, dedicated, and determined professionals committed to performing their tasks as members of a profession whose importance was steadily growing. They were also committed to becoming part of the larger community of psychiatrists not because of any yearning to belong to the "fraternity," as it were, but because it could provide a rich opportunity for growth and service to their own patients.

Some of the pioneer black American psychiatrists, and even a good number in more recent times, had to make strenuous efforts to become a part of the larger scientific community. One is appalled in attempting to count the costs of such efforts. Suppose, for example, that Solomon Carter Fuller, from the time he graduated from Boston University Medical School in 1897 to, say, 1917, could have given all his attention to pursuing his specialty in psychiatry instead of attempting to find a place in this country where he could get the necessary training. He would certainly have been able to expend all his energies on his work instead of attempting to find a place in Europe where he could study neuropathology and psychiatry. Happily, he found Munich a hospitable environment in which to engage in further study. The same experience was shared by many other black American psychiatrists, such as George Branch, Charles Prudhomme, Ernest Y. Williams, and Margaret Morgan Lawrence, all of whom in one way or another experienced difficulties in securing advanced training or experience in the field.

Ironies abound. White psychiatrists, surely more than most groups, should have been able to appreciate the importance of a healthy mental state for the pursuit of a highly specialized and difficult field. But they were often unyielding in their determination to keep blacks and women out of the field. They had to know the damage they could inflict on an individual or a group by their own intransigence. Yet they were loath to admit black American colleaguesinto the hospitals, clinics, or professional associations.

If they would do such a thing to their own colleagues merely because they were of a different race, one wonders whether this insensitivity was reflected in their dealings with their own black American patients. One wonders further, if one's mental health could possibly improve in such an environment.

If black American psychiatrists encountered serious problems in entering the profession in earlier years and if they have found some glitches along the way in their relationships with white colleagues, it can be said that they have "come of age" and that they now occupy a very important place in the mental health arena in this country. Black American psychiatric professionals no longer work exclusively at the small number of historically black medical schools but are scattered through the departments of psychiatry and related fields at many of the major U.S. medical colleges and facilities. They may be found in state departments of mental health and at the National Institute of Mental Health. They are in private practice and in academic medicine. Indeed, wherever problems of mental health are on the agenda, whether at the American Psychiatric Association or at some community group dealing with mental health, black American psychiatrists are present in ever-increasing numbers.

This book reflects the remarkable growth and influence of black American psychiatrists. The essays, covering virtually every possible area and reach of the field, provide an important tool not only for the professional but for the layperson as well. One cannot come away from this work without having gained a sense of what it was like to live through some tumultuous times. Nor can the reader fail to appreciate what the pioneers did and what the tireless and gifted professionals continue to do to improve the mental health of black communities and, indeed, the mental health of the nation.

—*John Hope Franklin*
  James B. Duke Professor Emeritus
  Department of History
  Duke University
  Durham, North Carolina

Preface

No doubt scores of colleagues have given thought to writing a history of the contributions that black psychiatrists have made to the multiple sections of our field and the field as a whole. In keeping with the black American oral tradition, some of us have talked about "how it used to be" as we recalled the spirited lectures of Justin Hope at Howard University College of Medicine and the wise teachings of Raphael Hernandez at Meharry Medical College. Howard alumni shared their knowledge about the personal sacrifices that E. Y. Williams had made in the development of the Department of Psychiatry at Howard, and alumni from both Howard and Meharry recalled their experiences as clinical students on a psychiatric rotation away from home base. A few of the current older generation had known the early pioneers, like Solomon Carter Fuller, S. O. Johnson, George Branch, Toussaint Tilden, Prince Barker, and Charles Prudhomme, all of whom (except Fuller) had been members of the staff of the Veterans Administration Hospital at Tuskegee.

Some of the older generation, who had their undergraduate and graduate education at predominately white institutions, shared their experiences—both positive and negative—during encounters of the past and more recently, too. Many of us, regardless of the site of our training, reflected on the assistance and support given to black trainees and young professionals by Viola Bernard.

Most of this history had been recorded only in the heads and hearts of individuals who had been intimately involved in it. Aware that some of our history was lost with the demise of colleagues from the "first generation," I became preoccupied with the idea of developing a written document. I was also aware of the significant contributions of our younger colleagues and wondered where this was being recorded, and by whom. But where to start?

The beginnings of this project had multiple roots, all pierced with one or several questions. As I gave thought to the content and the contributors, I focused on the possibility and my hope that historian John Hope Franklin would write the Foreword. Indeed, I am most pleased that he, one of my heroes, agreed to do so.

The selection of our name identification was not free of conflict. Most readers are aware of the several labels black Americans have been given (or have selected), including colored, Negro, Afro-American, African American, Black, Black American, black. During this struggle I conferred with colleagues in several fields. I chose to use the term *black*, which I believe is inclusive of all black people who reside in the United States.

It was my intention that the authors represent our leaders across generations and in different areas of our work. Regrettably, some colleagues declined for personal reasons. Fortunately, the greater number responded affirmatively and with expressions of keen interest.

Initially, I gave considerable thought to the matter of publishing—which publisher might be interested and the one from which black colleagues would welcome an "endorsement" by its publication of the volume. For a number of reasons, not the least important of which was the fact that I have been a member of the staff of the American Psychiatric Association for a number of years, I first approached the American Psychiatric Press (APPI). After some negotiations, which focused primarily on length, an agreement was reached and a contract signed. The designated number of pages served to limit the content.

The search for data was no easy task. Some authors circulated questionnaires to members who had been identified as devoting the greater percentage of their time in a particular area of our field. One coauthor circulated a questionnaire (pertaining to experiences in academe) to all the known black psychiatrists. Although responses were fewer in number than hoped for, considerable and significant information was obtained. Early on, other contributors and I announced the development of the volume at various professional meetings and requested that any pertinent information be forwarded to them. A notice about the effort and a request for information also appeared in a Black Psychiatrists of America (BPA) publication. Information was also sought from colleagues during telephone interviews and through perusals of numbers of volumes in the Black Studies section of the Martin Luther King Jr. Memorial Library in Washington, DC. Information was also garnered from several videotapes of black psychiatrists that were produced by Richard Fields during the time of his presidency of the BPA and from reviews of the oral histories of black psychiatrists that are housed in the library of the American Psychiatric Association.

Certainly, this volume is the work of many, many individuals. I am grateful to each and every contributor—not only the authors but to the many individuals (psychiatrists and nonpsychiatrists) who were willing to give their time to listen to my questions and to respond. I sincerely regret that personal circumstances accounted for the nonresponse from some of our colleagues. I do appreciate the responses of others and am especially appreciative of the assistance provided by William Baxter, former chief librarian at the American Psychiatric Association, and to his successor, Susan Heffner. I thank my colleague, Martin Booth, who read and commented on several manuscripts, and Ethel Taylor, who was most helpful in obtaining a commitment from Bonita Owens, who typed the manuscripts. I am indebted, too, to my sister, Joyce Jones, and my niece, Allison Winfield, who provided editorial assistance for several chapters. Each of my sisters, Frances Blackburn, Joyce Jones, and Sharon Dennis, is deserving of special thanks; they were readily available to listen to my complaints about the plight of an editor and to lend their support.

—Jeanne Spurlock, M.D.

PART I

Historical Reviews

CHAPTER 1

Early and Contemporary Pioneers

JEANNE SPURLOCK, M.D.

Biographical Sketches of a Sampling of Early Pioneers

Solomon Carter Fuller, M.D.

Identified as the first black psychiatrist in the United States, Solomon Carter Fuller, a native of Liberia, graduated from Livingston College (Salisbury, North Carolina). He pursued medical education at Boston University, from which he graduated in 1897. His professional training took place in an era that was studded with gains and losses for black Americans. Many Negroes, as black Americans were called then, had earned accolades for their achievements. Booker T. Washington founded Tuskegee Institute in 1881, and 1 year later, George Washington Williams published his two-volume book, *History of the Negro Race in America*. Daniel Hale Williams, M.D., performed the first open-heart surgical procedure in Chicago's Provident Hospital in 1893, and W. E. B. Du Bois earned his doctorate from Harvard University in 1895. The Civil Rights Act had been passed in 1875, but the Supreme Court voided much of the law in 1883 (Franklin 1976). The discriminatory practices that were prevalent in organized medicine led to the organization of the National Medical Association (NMA) in 1895.

Charles A. Pinderhughes, M.D., who had numerous contacts with Fuller, reported (personal communication) that Fuller received psychiatric training at Boston University, Long Island College Hospital, and Westborough State Hospital in Massachusetts between 1897 and 1901. For the next 2 years he worked at Westborough State Hospital as a clinician and pathologist. Desiring advanced training and unable to obtain a post in the United States,

Fuller explored the possibilities abroad. He succeeded in arranging a period of study (1904–1905) under Emil Kraepelin, Alois Alzheimer, Otto von Bollinger, and Hans Schmans at the University of Munich. Upon completion of his formal training, Fuller returned to the United States, where he established a career as a clinician, researcher, and educator. He served as a clinical psychiatrist and neurologist at Westborough State Hospital for 45 years and as a pathologist for 22 years of his tenure. For more than 30 years, he taught psychiatry, neurology, and neuropathology at Boston University School of Medicine. He retired as professor emeritus in 1937.

Fuller gained greater acceptance and recognition primarily as a neuropathologist, although he maintained an interest in and alertness for clinical work. In 1906, at the 62nd annual meeting of the American Psychiatric Association, he presented a paper, "A Study of the Neurofibrils in Dementia Paralytica, Dementia Senilis, Chronic Alcoholism, Cerebral Lues, and Microcephalic Idiocy." An expanded version of the paper was published in the *American Journal of Insanity*, now known as the *American Journal of Psychiatry*, the following year.

Recruitment of Black Psychiatrists for Tuskegee VA Hospital

In the early 1920s Fuller was approached by Michael O. Dumas, M.D., a member of the council of the National Medical Association, and John A. Kenney, M.D., the medical director of the John A. Andrew Memorial Hospital in Tuskegee, Alabama, to assist in the recruitment of black psychiatrists for Tuskegee Veterans Administration (VA) Hospital. This request followed a struggle that was embedded in the resistance of the Veterans Bureau to appointing black medical staff to the hospital that was developed for black veterans.[1] Fuller provided an orientation to psychiatry and some elementary training to three 1923 graduates of Boston medical schools. All of these young physicians—George Branche, S. O. Johnson, and Toussaint Tilden—later accepted staff positions at Tuskegee VA Hospital.

George Branche held several clinical posts at Tuskegee VA Hospital before his appointment as chief of clinical services in 1946. As indicated previously, he had received some psychiatric training during an externship at Boston Psychopathic Hospital in 1923. Early in 1927 (February 28–May 1)

---

1. This problem was resolved when President Harding responded affirmatively to a request forwarded by Tuskegee Institute's president, Dr. Robert R. Moton. The request: "Give Negro physicians an opportunity to qualify for service in the hospital through special civil service examinations" (Morais 1967, p. 114). In 1924, Dr. Joseph H. Ward, a black World War I veteran, was appointed the hospital's medical officer in chief.

Branche had additional formal training in neuropsychiatry at Bronx VA Hospital. Prior to his appointment as chief of the Neuropsychiatry Service at Tuskegee VA Hospital in 1927, Branche held a staff position for 4 years at the same hospital.

S(imon) O. Johnson pursued formal psychiatric training at Boston Psychopathic and Montefiore hospitals and received additional training at London National Hospital and Salpêtrière in Paris. Following his tenure at Tuskegee VA Hospital, Johnson accepted the post of superintendent of Lakin State Hospital (Lakin, West Virginia),where he succeeded in recruiting a number of black physicians to provide primary health care services. He apparently served as a significant role model in that several of these physicians, as noted below, went on to pursue formal training in psychiatry.

After graduating from Harvard University School of Medicine in 1923, Toussaint Tilden spent most of his career at Tuskegee in the areas of administrative and clinical psychiatry.

After the appointments of Branche, Johnson, and Tilden, other black psychiatrists worked at Tuskegee for varying periods. Prince Barker, Raphael Hernandez, Alan Percival Smith, and Charles Prudhomme were among those who had assignments at Tuskegee in the early years of blacks in psychiatry.

Raphael Hernandez, M.D.

A 1928 graduate of Meharry Medical College in Nashville, Tennessee, Hernandez pursued graduate education in neuropsychiatry and encephalography at Mason General Hospital in Brentwood, New York, and Hines VA Hospital (Illinois) and was certified in psychiatry and neurology. He also earned a law degree at Chicago Kent College of Law. Hernandez, a native of Puerto Rico, referred to himself as a "person of color" (L. C. Elam, personal communication, April 1995). He was multilingual, fluent in Spanish, English, French, Italian, and Portuguese. Long before Meharry developed its Department of Psychiatry, he was teaching psychiatry there. Hernandez served as chief of psychiatry-neurology services at the VA Hospital in San Juan (1947–1954) and chief of the neurology service at Tuskegee VA Hospital (1954–1956) and in 1956 was appointed chief of neurology-psychiatry and EEG services at the VA Hospital in Murfreesboro, Tennessee. In 1960 he was named director of the Negro section of the state hospital in Nashville. The racial discrimination that existed within the medical profession at that time is reflected in the words of a white colleague who wrote in support of Hernandez's membership application to the American Psychiatric Association:

I do not know personally of his publications since the Colored and White Medical Associations in the South are separate and his publications would not be printed in our State journal.

In attesting to his acumen, reference to racial separation was noted by another colleague.

I am very glad to say that he is one of the best informed colored men I have ever met, in neurology and psychiatry.

Ernest Y. Williams, M.D.

A native of Nevis, British West Indies, Williams came to the United States (in the early 1900s) slowly; that is, he had stopovers in St. Kitts, St. Thomas, and Puerto Rico before arriving in the United States, where he planned to attend college and graduate school. He had no particular interest in medicine during his childhood and adolescence; in fact, he had been an accomplished pianist and wanted to pursue a career in music. His father discouraged this interest, fearing financial insecurity. Following his father's advice he talked with an uncle, who was an engineer. When Williams came to the United States, his goal was to study engineering. In response to a question raised during an interview by Richard Fields, then the president of the Black Psychiatrists of America, about the onset of his interest in medicine, Williams said he "went into medicine to stay close to two people to whom I had loaned money." He explained that it was possible that if he was too far away, the borrowers would forget about the loan.

As a medical student at Howard University from 1926 to 1930, Williams served a clinical rotation at St. Elizabeths Hospital in Washington, D.C. One day, Williams's attention was directed to a radio broadcast of a game of baseball's World Series between the Detroit Tigers and the St. Louis Cardinals. A patient approached him and began naming the players on both teams; "we struck up a friendship," Williams later said. Afterward, Dr. Benjamin Karpman, a senior medical officer at St. Elizabeths, asked Williams if he had known the patient, adding that the patient had not talked to anyone in the 18 months of his hospital stay. The young medical student was thus assigned to take a complete history of the patient. Over a period of several days he wrote 57 pages of history. Impressed with the student's ability, the attending psychiatrist gave him another assignment—taking a history from an alcoholic female patient. This history was less extensive than that of the first patient (only 38 pages). Williams recalled that his history of this patient had been included in Karpman's book, *The Alcoholic Woman,* although Karpman made no reference to the fact that Williams had taken the history.

In 1931, the year after he was awarded the M.D. degree at Howard University, Williams won a 2-year fellowship in neuropsychiatry at Columbia University College of Physicians and Surgeons in New York City. Upon completion of the fellowship, which had apparently been orchestrated by Dr. Karpman, he returned to Howard University, where he was appointed to several posts (instructor, assistant professor, and associate professor) prior to his appointment as professor and head of the Department of Psychiatry in 1952. His ascent in academe and the development of the department was not free of difficulties, some thornier than others.

In the interview with Richard Fields referred to previously, Williams cited the struggles he experienced related to fund-raising. It was not unusual for him to use his personal funds (from a part-time enterprise as a realtor) to finance programs that were essential to the operation of the department. His recall of these personal contributions does not diminish the efforts that he directed to grant writing and the resultant successes—the awarding of funds. In 1939, a year before his appointment as chief of the division of neuropsychiatry in Freedmen's Hospital, he established a psychiatric service, which had grown to 24 beds by 1957. All-day clinics in neuropsychiatry were established in 1954. In 1955 he was successful in obtaining approval of a 3-year residency training program. The instruction provided by Williams and one of his chief associates, Justin Hope, M.D. (a member of the department from 1942 to 1948), served to trigger and reinforce the interest of a sizeable number of students in pursuing training in psychiatry.[2]

Charles Prudhomme, M.D.

After completing a psychiatry-neurology fellowship (University of Chicago, 1937–1938), Charles Prudhomme, a 1935 graduate of Howard University School of Medicine, applied for but was not accepted into formal training in psychiatry at St. Elizabeths Hospital. Charles Griffith, who had been responsible for planning the desegregation of the medical staff at Tuskegee

---

2. One of these students, Shirley Williams, M.D., followed in her father's footsteps. She too trained in neurology (Bellevue Hospital, New York City) and psychiatry (Henry Ford Hospital, Detroit). Since 1966, she has been the chief of Norwalk Hospital (Norwalk, Connecticut) Ambulatory Psychiatry. She retired from this position in 1998.

VA Hospital and was then reassigned as the medical director there, encouraged Prudhomme to accept an assignment as associate medical officer at Tuskegee VA Hospital. Prudhomme accepted the assignment in 1939 and remained there for $4\frac{1}{2}$ years before returning to Howard University, where he was an instructor in physiology in the medical school. He also held appointments as lecturer in the School of Social Work and staff psychiatrist at the University Health Service.

Prudhomme, who completed psychoanalytic training at the Washington Psychoanalytic Institute in 1956, is said to have been the first black American psychoanalyst. Often a victim of racial discrimination, he devoted a significant amount of time and energy during his professional career to working toward the elimination of racist practices. Some of his experiences as an activist are outlined in a chapter (Prudhomme and Musto 1973) in *Racism and Mental Health*. Following the desegregation of the armed forces, precipitated by President Truman's executive order in 1948, a group of black physicians and others met with the head of the Veterans Administration, General Omar Bradley, to discuss desegregating VA hospitals. Prudhomme was included in this meeting and in subsequent exchanges with the medical director, General Paul Hawley, and Winfred Overholser, superintendent of St. Elizabeths Hospital and the recently elected president of the American Psychiatric Association. Overholser expressed opposition to desegregation and indicated that such a move would not be in the best interest of patients. At noon on the second day of this 2-day meeting, General Bradley joined the group to report that he had received a telephone call from the White House. President Truman had ordered the desegregation of all VA hospitals.

The landmark school desegregation case, *Brown v. Board of Education of Topeka, Kansas* (1954), was another event of national note in which Prudhomme became involved as a psychiatrist. In response to a request from the team of lawyers based at Howard University, Prudhomme approached the leadership of the American Psychiatric Association to garner support for overturning school segregation. Specifically, he requested that the association file a brief amicus curiae "supporting the contention that separate educational facilities are not equal" (p. 47). The association leadership advised Prudhomme "to withdraw from involvement in the case and remain aloof from such a political issue" (p. 73).

Prudhomme is remembered for a number of distinguished firsts, including being the first black psychiatrist appointed (by the Chief Judge of the U.S. District Courts) to the Mental Health Commission, which had been charged with reviewing the involuntary hospitalization of the mentally ill in the District of Columbia. A little-known fact about Prudhomme is the role he played in professional baseball. Before desegregation of the sport, he was a pitcher for the Kansas City Monarchs of the Negro Leagues.

Administrative and Clinical Psychiatrists: A Sampling of Early and Contemporary Pioneers

E. Pentoka Henry, M.D., who completed undergraduate medical education at the University of West Tennessee in 1928, spent most of his career at Taft State Hospital (originally known as the State Hospital for the Negro Insane), where he held various positions prior to his appointment as medical superintendent in 1938. The hospital was located in Taft, Oklahoma, one of several black towns that were established after the Civil War. Walter Adams, a 1928 graduate of Howard University School of Medicine, completed psychiatry training at Boston Psychopathic Hospital and settled in Chicago. He established a psychiatry clinic at Provident Hospital and a private practice.

As noted previously, S. O. Johnson apparently served as an influential role model to some primary care physicians who worked under his tutelage when he was superintendent of Lakin State Hospital. It was at Lakin that their interest in psychiatry was generated or reinforced. Included in this group were Eugene Youngue Jr., Mildred Mitchell-Bateman, Kathryn Rainbow-Earhart, James Bell, Zelda Bowie-Elder, Luther Robinson, and Dorothea Simmons. For a brief period, January 1, 1946, to the end of February 1947, Youngue served as a staff physician and then as acting superintendent at Lakin. He moved on to pursue formal psychiatric training at Homer G. Phillips Hospital in St. Louis (1947–1949) and Menninger School of Psychiatry and Winter VA Hospital (1949–1950). Bell served as clinical director (1948–1951) at Lakin prior to psychiatry training (general and child) at the Menninger School (1953–1957).

Upon completion of a psychiatric residency (1952–1955) at Menninger School of Psychiatry and Winter VA Hospital, Mildred Mitchell-Bateman, M.D., returned to Lakin, where she held the post of clinical director. In 1958 she was promoted to superintendent. She resigned from this post in 1960 when she accepted a supervisory position at the West Virginia Department of Mental Health. In 1962 she was named commissioner of this department (the first black to be appointed commissioner of a Department of Mental Health), a post she held for 15 years. In 1977 she accepted an appointment to chair the department of psychiatry at Marshall University School of Medicine. (A segment of her work is described in chapter 12 in this book.)

Kathryn Rainbow-Earhart succeeded Mitchell-Bateman as superintendent at Lakin in 1960. Previously she had held the posts of staff physician (1954–1959) and clinical director (1959–1960). She left Lakin to pursue psychiatric training at Menninger School of Psychiatry. Upon completion, in 1965, she accepted a staff position at the State Hospital in Topeka.

Robert Walden served as superintendent of Lakin from 1962 to 1965. Previously he had been acting clinical director at Taft State Hospital (Oklahoma) from 1950 to 1953, staff physician at Tuskegee VA Hospital from 1955 to 1957, and staff psychiatrist at the VA Hospital in Pittsburgh from 1960 to 1962. After his tenure at Lakin, Walden moved to the Midwest, where he was in community psychiatry in Michigan and Ohio, then joined the faculty at the Medical College of Ohio, Toledo, in 1968.

Luther Robinson's 2-year appointment (1947–1949) was followed by his induction into the army and an assignment (primarily as a psychiatrist) in the Far East. After his discharge, he received some formal training in psychiatry at Freedmen's and St. Elizabeths hospitals. He was the first black physician accepted for psychiatric training at St. Elizabeths and credits his acceptance to being in the right place at the right time in history. He accepted a staff position as a medical officer in 1955, then served as acting superintendent (December 1969–June 1972) and superintendent (June 1972–July 1975). Prior to his formal retirement in 1994, Robinson was acting chairperson of the Department of Psychiatry at Howard University College of Medicine.

Beginning in the early 1960s, Crownsville State Hospital[3] in Maryland was another psychiatric facility that provided career and training opportunities for black psychiatrists and residents. In 1963 the State of Maryland, under the leadership of Isadore Tuerek, M.D., then director of the Mental Hygiene Administration, desegregated the Mental Hospital System. Before 1963 Crownsville State Hospital had been the only state facility to serve black mentally ill patients. Clifton T. Perkins Hospital had been established in 1960 as the state's hospital for the criminally insane. At the time of its opening, Perkins was fully integrated.

---

3. The author is grateful to Dr. John M. Hamilton for providing historical information about this facility.

In 1965 Tuerek appointed Drs. George McKenzie Phillips and John M. Hamilton as superintendents of Perkins and Crownsville, respectively. Both men had had some earlier association with Crownsville. Hamilton had completed the first 2 years of his psychiatric residency at Crownsville before being accepted at the University of Maryland in 1957 for his final year of training. He noted that this appointment, as the first black resident in psychiatry, was accomplished not without a struggle. Phillips, who had completed his residency training at Howard University's Freedmen's Hospital, had been appointed to the post of clinical director at Crownsville in 1959.

James Peal held the position of assistant director of Michigan State Department of Mental Health from 1964 to 1967. Other black psychiatrists appointed to state posts included Audrey Worrell as commissioner in Connecticut, 1981; and Harold W. Jordan as assistant commissioner, 1971, and commissioner, 1975, in Tennessee. Tony Gore was appointed senior deputy commissioner/medical director of the South Carolina Department of Mental Health in 1986. In 1992, Walter Shervington took leave from an academic post at Louisiana State University School of Medicine to accept the position of assistant secretary of the Office of Mental Health, Department of Health and Hospitals, State of Louisiana. Roy Wilson became commissioner of the Missouri Department of Mental Health in 1995. The first psychiatrist since 1979 and the first black American to be appointed to the post, Wilson was selected from a field of 82 applicants. June Jackson Christmas and Billy Jones were each appointed commissioner of Mental Health and Mental Retardation and Alcoholism Services of New York City at different times—Christmas in 1972 and Jones in 1990. Jones was also named, in 1992, the president of Health and Hospital Corporation in New York City (an election brought about the defeat of the incumbent mayor and Jones' term of office was interrupted).

Other administrative positions held by black psychiatrists include posts within the United States Department of State, the Department of Health and Human Services, the Association of American Medical Colleges, and the American Psychiatric Association. Currently (1998), Esther Roberts holds the position of Regional Psychiatrist, London Medical Evacuation Center, U.S. Department of State. Previously, she was director of mental health programs in the Office of Medical Services of the Department of State, as well as a deputy assistant secretary in the same office and had completed assignments in Thailand, Mexico, and France (based in Paris). Prior to his appointment in 1988 as vice president, Division of Minority Health, Education and Prevention of the Association of American Medical Colleges, Herbert Nickens served as the director of the Office on Minority

Health, Department of Health and Human Services. Appointees to administrative posts at the American Psychiatric Association are identified under that heading later in this chapter.

Medical Education

As indicated earlier, E. Y. Williams, M.D., who spent most of his professional career at Howard University, organized the Department of Psychiatry there and was appointed head of the department in 1952. In 1968 he was succeeded by Edward Rickman, who was followed in 1973 by Walter Bradshaw in an acting position. The following year (1974) Samuel C. Bullock was appointed to head the department. Bullock was succeeded by James L. Collins in 1979. When Collins resigned in 1986 to resume his military career, Luther D. Robinson was appointed acting head. He held that position until 1989, at which time Maxie C. Maultsby Jr. was appointed to head the department. When Maultsby took a sabbatical leave in 1995, Walter Bland was appointed acting chairperson.

In Chapter 4 of this book, Lloyd Elam recounts his experiences of being recruited, during the last year (1960–1961) of his psychiatric residency training, to chair the developing Department of Psychiatry at Meharry Medical College. Subsequent to Elam's appointment as acting dean and before his appointment as president of the College, the author was appointed (in 1968) to chair the department. She was succeeded by William Coopwood as acting chairperson and then by William Grier and Harold Jordan.

J. Alfred Cannon and Dewitt Alfred earned and accepted leadership roles in the psychiatry departments they headed at the two newest black medical schools—Charles Drew Post Graduate Medical School in Los Angeles (established in 1970) and Morehouse School of Medicine in Atlanta (established in 1978). Each was assisted in his work by colleagues in the respective local communities. Ellis Toney, Gloria Keyes, George Mallory, Florence Douglas, Amos Davis, Rose Jenkins, and Anna Smith, all psychiatrists, are known to have made significant contributions to the development and growth of the department at Drew. Mallory also recalled the major contributions of Hiawatha Harris, director of Central City Mental Health Center, and James Jones, who headed the Kendren Mental Health Center. The development of Drew Post Graduate School of Medicine and its teaching facility, Martin Luther King Jr. Hospital, occurred during the height of the Civil Rights movement in the 1960s and at a time in history when there was a focus on community involvement and service. Following his tenure as the head of psychiatry, Cannon chaired the Department of International Medicine and then made a move to Zimbabwe. Cannon's successors include Frank W. Hayes (1979–1982), who headed the Department of Psychiatry at the Uniformed Services University School of Medicine (1976–1979); and Claudewell Thomas (1982–1993), who had chaired the Department of Psychiatry at the University of New Jersey College of Medicine and Dentistry from 1973 to 1979. Clinical psychologist Joan Cooper and psychiatrist Frank E. Pinder were appointed interim cochairpersons in 1993. From 1977 to 1979 three individuals, Gloria Keyes, M.D., George Mallory, M.D., and Jocelyn White, Ph.D., were appointed (at different times) to serve as interim chair.

Dewitt Alfred was appointed to head the department at Morehouse in 1978. A report of the school's early history (Alfred, personal communication, 1995) parallels that of Meharry in that the greater number of faculty held full-time appointments at another school. In fact, for the first 5 years (1978–1983), classes for junior medical students were held at Emory College of Medicine. Several psychiatrists, including Iverson Bell (director of training), John Gaston, Gail Mattox, and Quentin Ted Smith, played key roles in the operation of the department, which received accreditation for residency training in 1990.

None of the four departments was immune to difficulties related to recruiting and retaining faculty, nor to the multiple problems that stemmed from insufficient funding. Williams, Elam, Cannon, Alfred, and their successors are to be commended for their efforts and range of contributions to our field.

In addition to Frank Hayes's and Claudewell Thomas's appointments to chair departments of psychiatry at predominately white schools, note is made of Donald Williams's appointment at Michigan State University College of Human Medicine. Williams chaired the psychiatry department from 1985 to 1989.

Academicians who pioneered at predominately white medical colleges include Drs. Chester Pierce (University of Oklahoma and Harvard); Charles Pinderhughes (Boston University, Harvard, and Tufts); James Curtis and Bruce Ballard (Cornell); June Jackson Christmas, Elizabeth Davis, and Margaret Morgan Lawrence (Columbia); Charles Wilkinson (University of Missouri); Robert Bragg (Harvard and University of Miami); Claire Assue (University of Indiana); Alvin Poussaint (Tufts and Harvard); Andre Tweed (Loma Linda); Ellis Toney (University of Southern California); Yvonne Ferguson and Gloria Johnson Powell (UCLA); Mildred Mitchell-Bateman

(Women's Medical College); Veva Zimmerman (New York University); William Womack (University of Washington); Robert Walden (Medical College of Ohio, Toledo); Roderick Charles (University of Buffalo); Mae McMillan (Baylor); Frances Jones Bonner (Boston University and Harvard); Jeanne Spurlock (University of Illinois, Chicago); James Comer, Ezra Griffith, and Donald Williams (Yale); Samuel Bullock (Temple and University of Pennsylvania); Gloria Onque (University of Pittsburgh); James Ralph (Johns Hopkins); and Billy Jones and Phyllis Harrison Ross (New York Medical College).

Clare Assue is believed to have been the first black psychiatrist appointed director of a psychiatric training program; she was named to this post at Indiana University School of Medicine in 1979. Several black psychiatrists have held or currently hold the position of associate dean in predominately white medical schools. Included in this group are James Curtis (appointed at Cornell in 1969), Alvin Poussaint at Harvard, James Comer at Yale, Veva Zimmerman at New York University, Billy Jones at New York Medical College, Leonard Lawrence at the University of Texas in San Antonio, and Bruce Ballard at Cornell. Charles Wilkinson held the post of assistant dean of curriculum (1971–1980) and associate dean for development (1980–1983) at the University of Missouri (Kansas City). A detailed account of the roles and work of black American academicians is outlined in Chapter 7, "Black Psychiatrists and Academia."

The Civil Rights Movement

Black psychiatrists were involved in various aspects of the movement. Charles Wilkinson, M.D., assumed a leadership role when he developed a proposal to obtain funding to support a series of meetings with several black psychiatrists (including Hugh Butts, Elizabeth Davis, Charles Pinderhughes, Lloyd Elam, William Tompkins, Chester Pierce, Alfred Cannon, Jeanne Spurlock, and James Comer) and neurologist Calvin Calhoun. Under Wilkinson's leadership, the group identified and scrutinized the various psychological ramifications of the Civil Rights movement on groups of black Americans and explored ways and means to enhance the positives and attenuate the negatives. Attention was also directed to the demands for changes within organized psychiatry and selected federal agencies. A new organization, the Black Psychiatrists of America (BPA), grew out of this effort. Although an autonomous body, the membership included black psychiatrists who were members of the National Medical Association and the American Psychiatric Association.

At a national level, Alvin Poussaint was the most visible black psychiatrist who was a full-time activist in the Movement. After completing psychiatric training in 1965, he accepted the post of southern field director of the Medical Committee for Human Rights (the medical arm of the Civil Rights Movement) in Jackson, Mississippi. His experiences and conclusions, which he outlined in his early publications (Poussaint 1966, 1968), remain pertinent to contemporary interracial relations. Drawing from their clinical experiences, William Grier and Price Cobbs (1968) wrote *Black Rage,* which became a best-seller in the late 1960s and early 1970s, although some of their conclusions were challenged by some black colleagues (Butts 1969, Spurlock 1971).

In the early 1970s a small group of black psychiatrists (Charles Prudhomme, Charles Pinderhughes, Jeanne Spurlock, Claudewell Thomas, James Comer, Gloria Johnson Powell, and Chester Pierce) were active participants in a series of seminars, supported by the Maurice Falk Medical Foundation, that focused on the impact of racism on the mental health of blacks in the United States. A modification of the formal presentations was published in *Racism and Mental Health* (Willie, Kramer, and Brown 1973).

In this era the publications of a number of black psychiatrists (Harrison and Butts 1970; Jones et al. 1970; Pinderhughes 1966, 1968, 1969; Spurlock 1973; Thomas and Comer 1973) focused on the impact of racism on the mental health of black people in the United States. The Jones et al. (1970) reference reflects the untoward experiences of black residents who trained in predominately white programs.

During this period many of the presentations at meetings of psychiatric societies also focused on the ramifications of racism on the mental health of black Americans. Standing-room-only attendance was common at many sessions of the National Medical Association's annual meetings. Crowd-drawing titles included the following: "White Psychiatrists' Racism in Referral Practices to Black Psychiatrists" (Phyllis Harrison-Ross and Hugh Butts), "The Negro Psyche: Fact, Fiction and Fantasy" (Alyce Gullattee), "The Impact of the Black Identity Crisis on Community Psychiatry" (Sidney Jenkins), "The Cress Theory of Color Confrontation and Racism—White Supremacy" (Frances Cress Welsing), and "Psychological and Physiological Origins of Racism and Other Social Discrimination" (Charles A. Pinderhughes).

Leadership in National Professional Organizations

National Medical Association (NMA)

In the very early years of the NMA, psychiatrists met with neurologists and neurosurgeons within the administrative structure of the Section on Neuropsychiatry, and the leadership rotated among the three groups. In the early 1980s the neurologists and neurosurgeons, who had increased in numbers (as had the psychiatrists), petitioned to form a separate neurology/neurosurgery section. At that time the Section on Psychiatry and Behavioral Science was named.

S. O. Johnson, who chaired the Section on Neuropsychiatry from 1953 to 1959, was succeeded by Herbert (Red) Erwin, who served until 1962. Eugene (Gene) Youngue was appointed to the position in 1963; Jeanne Spurlock succeeded him in 1965. Subsequent chairpersons included Jaime Smith é Incas, Walter Shervington, George A. Mallory, Carol A. Leal, Carl C. Bell, Robert T. M. Phillips, Anne M. Bell, Ramona Davis, and Shirley Marks.

During his leadership George Mallory succeeded in obtaining funding (from the Mead Johnson Pharmaceutical Division of Mead Johnson & Company) for the development of the E. Y. Williams, M.D. Clinical Scholars of Distinction Awards honoring senior psychiatrists and residents. Early in his tenure as chair of the section, Robert T. M. Phillips organized and obtained funding (from the Dista Division of Eli Lilly Company and the Upjohn Company) for the Chester M. Pierce, M.D., Sc.D. Resident and Medical Student Research Symposium. Some outstanding work has been presented by the recipients of each of the awards.

Members of the section have been pleased to recognize psychiatry colleagues who have been elected to NMA executive offices. Leonard Lawrence was the first psychiatrist to be elected to the presidency (1993). Walter Shervington has held the offices of Speaker of the House of Delegates (1969–1991) and chair of the board of trustees (1995). Shirley Marks was elected Speaker of the House of Delegates in 1993. In 1998 Shervington held the office of president-elect.

American Psychiatric Association

Before 1969, when the leadership of the newly formed Black Psychiatrists of America directed efforts to widening opportunities for black psychiatrists in leadership positions, several black psychiatrists had been visible and active members of the Assembly of District Branches. Chester Pierce, John Anderson, Mildred Mitchell-Bateman, and George Mallory had been elected representatives of their respective branches (Oklahoma, Central Missouri, West Virginia, and Southern California). Mallory was elected to the post of recorder of the Assembly for a 1-year term in 1975; he was defeated in the 1976 election for speaker.

In 1969 the board of trustees responded affirmatively to several demands from the Executive Committee of the Black Psychiatrists of America. Immediate action was taken; the Ad Hoc Committee of Black Psychiatrists was formed, with Chester Pierce appointed chair. The nominating committee selected Charles Prudhomme as a candidate for the vice presidency. In spite of protests of a group of members based in the Washington, D.C., area, Prudhomme's name was placed on the ballot, and he won the election. Jeanne Spurlock, one of three candidates for that post in 1972, was defeated. Mildred Mitchell-Bateman and June Jackson Christmas were elected vice president in 1973 and 1974, respectively. Mitchell-Bateman's defeat for the presidency in 1976 provoked several questions among the membership: were members not ready for a black woman, or any woman or any black person, in the top post; or did overwhelming numbers view her opponent, Robert Gibson, as more knowledgeable about issues of particular importance (e.g., insurance coverage) at that time? Charles Wilkinson was twice elected treasurer (1976 and 1978) but was defeated by Daniel Freedman in the 1981 presidential election. Wilkinson's interest in working for and within the organizational structure continued, and he made significant contributions to the components to which he was appointed (e.g., the editorial board of the *American Journal of Psychiatry,* 1980–1988, and the Council on Internal Organization, which he chaired in 1991).

As a trustee at large, a 3-year post to which he was elected in 1974, Charles Pinderhughes was unswerving in addressing and upholding statements and proposals that related particularly to the mental health of minority populations. To this end, he objected strongly to the board of trustees' reversal of its endorsement of the United Nations Draft Program for a Decade of Action to Combat Racism and Racial Discrimination, and voiced strong support of the Resolution Against Apartheid.

Walter Bradshaw, chairperson of the Committee of Black Psychiatrists, alerted the board of trustees to charges of racial discrimination in the psychiatric service system in South Africa and suggested that APA take action to denounce this alleged policy. Smith, Mitchell & Co., a private group that orchestrated the provision of services at the public psychiatric hospitals in South Africa, denied the charges and invited an inspection team of two APA psychiatrists to investigate the charges. The board of trustees accepted the invitation (which included the offer to reimburse transportation costs and lodging) and committed funds to cover the cost of an additional two inspectors. Jack Weinberg, then president of the APA, appointed Alan Stone (then president-elect), Charles Pinderhughes, and Jeanne Spurlock to the team. Weinberg joined the group as an observer-participant. The report of the 1978 visit was published in *American Journal of Psychiatry* (volume 136, number 23) in 1979.

The Committee of Black Psychiatrists, under the leadership of Bruce Ballard, addressed the matter of psychiatric services for Haitian refugees detained at the U.S. Naval Base at Guantanamo Bay in Cuba. These discussions led to a recommendation to establish a liaison between the National Institute of Mental Health (NIMH) Cuban/Haitian Mental Health Unit and the APA Central Office to identify areas of cooperation between NIMH and APA in providing psychiatric care to Haitian refugees. The committee also addressed psychiatric services for black Americans, especially relating to misdiagnosis and deficient treatment measures. Walter Bradshaw developed a course, "Improving Skills for Psychiatric Treatment of Black Patients," for attendees of the APA annual meeting for three successive years (1981–1983). The author conducted a similar course in 1992 and 1993.

The idea for increasing the participation of black psychiatrists in the Assembly of District Branches grew out of discussions held by the Committee of Black Psychiatrists. In the mid-1970s Walter Bradshaw and Andrea Delgado, chairperson and vice chairperson of the committee, began negotiations with the leadership of the assembly and district branch representatives to establish an infrastructure that would assure the membership and participation of black and other minority psychiatrists. The proposed structure, which was approved by the governing body, permitted the organization of minority caucuses that would each elect a representative and deputy representative to act on their behalf during the meetings of the assembly. Richard Dudley, Donna Norris, Gilbert Parks, Yvonne Ferguson, John Gaston, and Freda Lewis-Hall were elected (at different times) representative or deputy representative of the Black Caucus. Carl Bell, Yvonne Ferguson, and John Gaston were elected president of the caucus.

William Womack and Donna Norris were elected to midlevel posts in the assembly, as representative and deputy representative of their respective districts (Washington State and the area of New England and eastern Canada). Norris was also elected a representative (to the assembly) of the Massachusetts Psychiatric Society and in 1996 was elected recorder of the assembly. In 1997 she held the office of speaker-elect.

The APA has recognized the achievements of a number of black psychiatrists in the presentations of awards. In 1985 Prudhomme was presented with the Distinguished Service Award. The Nominating Committee that submitted Prudhomme's name for this recognition called attention to his distinguished service to APA and American Psychiatry and his commitment to excellence in patient care. He was also a recipient of the Solomon Carter Fuller, M. D. Award, given to a black American in recognition of his or her work in promoting the mental health of black Americans. Other psychiatrists who have received the Fuller Award include Charles Pinderhughes, Chester Pierce, Gloria Johnson Powell, Luther Robinson, Jeanne Spurlock, James Comer, Dewitt Alfred, June Jackson Christmas, and Alvin Poussaint. Comer was also the recipient (1989) of the Agnes Purcell McGavin Award for outstanding contributions to the preventive aspects of emotional disorders of childhood, and was given a Special Presidential Commendation Award in 1990. Spurlock received the McGavin Award in 1989, a Special Presidential Commendation Award in 1992, and the Distinguished Service Award in 1996.

Four black psychiatrists were appointed to the APA staff. In 1972 Elvin Mackey was appointed by then medical director Walter Barton to direct the Minority Group Program. After Mackey's resignation, which was effective in 1974, Jeanne Spurlock was appointed (by Dr. Barton, who was soon to retire, and his successor, Melvin Sabshin) to expand the Minority Group Program and develop the Office of Minority Affairs. Subsequent appointments (by the medical director) included John M. Hamilton (1988) and Robert T. M. Phillips (1993). As the director of the Office of Minority/National Affairs (1974–1991) Spurlock was also the administrator of the APA/NIMH Minority Fellowship Program and collaborated with Harold Alan Pincus (director of the Office of Research) to develop the Program for Minority Research Training in Psychiatry (PMRTP). During Spurlock's tenure, over two hundred residents participated in the program. Hamilton served for 3 years as the director of the Office of Psychiatric Services; in that position he was responsible for direct management of the peer review and quality assurance program and edited two printings of the APA's *Peer Review Manual* and a book, *Peer Review Prelude and Promise*. The latter publication chronicles the association's history and outlook regarding medical review and quality assurance. Phillips held three positions simultaneously—director of the Office of Minority/National Affairs, director of the Office of Psychiatric Services, and director of the Office of Economic Affairs. Spurlock, Hamilton, and Phillips also held the title of deputy medical director.

Black Psychiatrists of America (BPA)

As noted earlier, BPA grew out of the efforts of a small group of black psychiatrists during the height of the Civil Rights Movement. The organization's birth took place in May 1969 at a caucus of black psychiatrists who were attending the annual meeting of the American Psychiatric Association. An account of BPA's history noted that "it was born to be action oriented" (Pierce 1973, p. 526). Chester Pierce and J. Alfred Cannon were elected chairman and vice chairman. James Comer and Hiawatha Harris were appointed to assist Pierce and Cannon in developing a list of resolutions and demands, some of which, upon approval of the BPA membership, were to be presented to the APA board of trustees. For the most part, the board responded affirmatively to the demands, which centered on changes in the organizational structure that would allow for increased and significant participation of black psychiatrists in the deliberations and operation of the APA. The Ad Hoc Committee of Black Psychiatrists (subsequently transformed into a permanent body) was established immediately. Chester Pierce, who was appointed to chair the committee, was authorized to participate in the proceedings (without a vote) of the board. In 1970, the APA executive committee acted on another demand and approved the employment of a black psychiatrist to direct the Minority Group Program. Elvin Mackey, on leave from the University of California, Irvine, occupied this post for 2 years (1972–1974).

Early efforts of the BPA leadership extended beyond the APA. Negotiations with NIMH and activities related to the American Board of Psychiatry and Neurology (ABPN) are illustrative. James Comer took a leadership role in negotiating with NIMH to develop a Center for Minority Group Mental Health Programs. In 1971 James Ralph was appointed chief of the center. The election of Chester Pierce to the board of directors of the ABPN exemplified another success of BPA's advocacy. BPA members who were elected to the presidency after Pierce's tenure were J. Alfred Cannon, James Comer, Charles Wilkinson, Phyllis Harrison-Ross, Carl Drake Jr., Billy E. Jones, Andrea K. Delgado, Ezra E. H. Griffith, Richard A. Fields, Thelissa Harris, Isaac Slaughter, William B. Lawson, Ramona Davis, and Altha Stewart. During her tenure as chair of the Program Committee, Delgado instituted a transcultural seminar that has become an annual event. These symposia, which have been held in a different Caribbean country each year, have attracted a broad representation of presenters and audience.

Under the leadership of Harrison-Ross, chair of the Program Committee, a 21-day scientific program recognizing the 25th anniversary of the founding of the BPA was held in New York City in March 1994. The theme, "The Black Psychiatrist into the 21st Century: Strengthening our Evolving Skills in Working with the Black Family and the Black Child," allowed for presentations of a variety of papers. The event provided an opportunity for participants to review the history of the BPA; identify new goals; and learn about new research, clinical, and educational efforts of the members. Two generations of black psychiatrists attended—the founding members and younger colleagues, some of whom had not yet completed formal training.

Early Contributors to Other National Professional Organizations

Early contributors to the Group for the Advancement of Psychiatry (GAP) included Charles Prudhomme, Charles Pinderhughes, and Rutherford (Rusty) Stevens. The latter two were members of the Committee on Social Issues, which published *Psychiatric Aspects of School Desegregation* (1957). Prudhomme had been invited to serve on the Committee on the College Student. James Bell worked with the Committee on Child Psychiatry, and Mildred Mitchell-Bateman and Lloyd Elam contributed to the work of the Committee on Public Education. Jeanne Spurlock served on the Committee on Adolescence and the Committee on Medical Education before transferring to the status of contributing member in the mid-1970s. Andrea Delgado was elected to the board of directors for a 2-year term (1978–1980). She established the Committee on Cultural Psychiatry and served as its chair until her untimely death in 1984. Charles Wilkinson was elected to the board of governors for two terms (1976–1980) and twice as treasurer (1983 and 1985). He was president-elect at the time of his death in 1992.

The multidisciplinary structure and the multicultural interests and efforts of the American Orthopsychiatry Association (AOA) attracted numbers of black psychiatrists to the AOA vineyards. Chester Pierce was elected to the presidency in 1983. James Comer, who chaired the Council on Problems of Minority Groups (1969–1971), also made significant contributions.

June Jackson Christmas's interest and work in the public sector carried over to her membership in the American Public Health Association. Certainly, her multiple efforts and sound contributions were applauded by members when she was elected president for the 1979–1980 term.

Early in the history of the American Academy of Child Psychiatry (later renamed the American Academy of Child and Adolescent Psychiatry), membership was by invitation. James Bell's and Jeanne Spurlock's invitation's to membership were approved in the mid-1960s. In 1967 Spurlock was elected to the council for a 2-year term and as secretary for 2 years in 1975. William Womack (in 1985), Marilyn Benoit (in 1984), and Harry Wright (in 1997) were also elected to the council. As their membership numbers increased, black psychiatrists were represented on a range of committees, but a greater number were active (by choice) on the Committee on Ethnic and Racial Issues. Four were appointed to chair committees: Jeanne Spurlock, Private Practice, 1967–1969; Leonard Lawrence, Membership Committee, 1983–1989; William Womack (appointed in 1991), Homosexual Issues; Marilyn Benoit (appointed in 1994), Child Abuse and Neglect. In 1997 Benoit was elected secretary.

Summary

The preceding text provides only sketches of the contributions of black psychiatrists who clearly were and are pioneers—early and contemporary—in the world of our profession. Even so, it reflects rich segments of history that had been known to only a few in our field. In the chapters that follow, accounts of the contributions of black psychiatrists in various subspecialties and different workplaces broaden the picture of the contributions of black psychiatrists to American psychiatry. Contemporary issues related to black psychiatrists and consumers are addressed in the final chapter.

References

Butts HF: White racism: Its origins, institutions and the implications for professional mental health practice. Int J Psychiatry 8(6):914–928, 1969

Comer JP: White racism: Its root, form and function. Am J Psychiatry 126(6):802–806, 1969

Committee on Social Issues: Psychiatric Aspects of School Desegregation. New York, Group for the Advancement of Psychiatry, 1957

Franklin JH: A brief history. In The Black American Reference Book. Edited by Smythe MM. Englewood Cliffs, NJ: Prentice-Hall, 1976, pp 1–89

Fuller SC: A study of the neurofibrils in dementia paralytica, dementia senilis, chronic alcoholism, cerebral lues and microcephalic idiocy. American Journal of Insanity 63:415–468, 1907

Grier WH, Cobbs PM: Black Rage. New York, Basic Books, 1968

Harrison P and Butts HF: White psychiatrists' racism in referral practice to black psychiatrists. J Nat Med Assoc 62:278–282

Jones BE, Lightfoot OB, Palmer D, et al: Problems of black psychiatric residents in white training institutions. Am J Psychiatry 127(6):798–803, 1970

Morais HM: The History of the Negro in Medicine. New York, Publishers, 1967

Pierce CM: The formation of the black psychiatrists of America. In Racism and Mental Health. Edited by Willie CV, Kramer BM, Brown BS. Pittsburgh, PA, University of Pittsburgh Press, 1973, pp 525–579

Pinderhughes CA: Pathogenic social structure: A prime target for preventive psychiatric intervention. J Nat Med Assoc 56(5):424–429, 1966

Pinderhughes CA: The psychodynamics of dissent: A clinical appraisal with emphasis on racial activists, in The Dynamics of Dissent. Edited by Masserman J. New York, Grune and Stratton, 1968, pp 56–81

Pinderhughes CA: Understanding black power: processes and proposals. Am J Psychiatry 125:1552–1557

Pinderhughes CA: Psychological and physiological origins of racism and other social discrimination. J Nat Med Assoc 63(1):25–29, 1971

Pinderhughes CA: The origins of racism. Int J Psychiatry 8: 914–941, 1979

Poussaint AF: The stresses of the white female worker in the civil rights movement in the South. Am J Psychiatry 123(4):401–407,1966

Poussaint AF: Black Power: A failure for integration within the civil rights movements. Arch Gen Psychiatry 18(4):385–391, 1968

Prudhomme C, Musto DF: Historical perspectives on mental health and racism in the United States, in Racism and Mental Health. Edited by Willie CV, Kramer BM, Brown BS. Pittsburgh, PA, University of Pittsburgh Press, 1973, pp 3–57

Spurlock J: A reappraisal of the role of black women. J Nat Assoc of Private Psychiatric Hospitals 3(3):8–17, 1971

Spurlock J: Some consequences of racism for children. In Racism and Mental Health. Edited by Willie CU, Kramer BM, Brown BS. Pittsburgh, PA: University of Pittsburgh Press, 1973, pp 147–163

Thomas CS, Comer JP: Racism and mental health services. In Racism and Mental Health. Edited by Willie CV, Kramer BM, Brown BS. Pittsburgh, PA: University of Pittsburgh Press, 1973, pp 165–181

CHAPTER 2

Development of a Department of Psychiatry in a General Hospital

ELIZABETH B. DAVIS, M.D.

The Beginnings

The Department of Psychiatry of the Harlem Hospital Center was established in the early 1960s during a period of massive reorganization and upgrading of care in the New York City municipal hospital system. In earlier decades the 21 city hospitals had had high medical standards. Both attending and house staff appointments were competitive and in demand. By the 1950s those municipal hospitals staffed by medical schools were still functioning at acceptable levels, but the volunteer physician system serving nonaffiliated hospitals had collapsed. A crisis in care and education had developed in the hospitals that had depended on a voluntary attending staff.

In February 1959, Mayor Robert F. Wagner appointed the Commission on Health Services to advise him. The commission's findings, of grave proportions, were reported during the summer of 1960 (Symposium on the Hospitals of New York City, 1961). In short order a national ruling was enforced banning foreign-trained house staff from patient care if they had not passed the examination given by the Educational Commission for Foreign Medical Graduates (ECFMG). The consequences of this for Harlem Hospital, specifically, were summarized in a report (Trussell 1962) to the New

York Academy of Medicine. Trussell noted that the ban occurred at a time of harsh weather conditions and a high accident rate in a community that made extensive use of emergency room services. An extremely distressful patient care situation developed.

Inpatient psychiatric services among the 21 municipal hospitals were limited to four institutions, with Bellevue Hospital serving as receiving hospital for all of the borough of Manhattan. At Harlem Hospital, some clinic services were directed by Dr. Harold Ellis, who was assisted by dedicated, but too few, personnel. The other major psychiatric function there was to sedate and restrain psychotic patients for transfer to Bellevue, where most were committed to a state hospital. Follow-up resources in Harlem were grossly inadequate.

In response to a press exposé of conditions at the Kings County Center psychiatric service (the receiving hospital for the borough of Brooklyn), a blue-ribbon panel, chaired by Dr. Lawrence Kolb (then chairman of the Department of Psychiatry at Columbia University), was appointed. During its investigation, the Kolb committee asked Mayor Wagner to tour Bellevue Hospital with his Commissioner of Hospitals, Dr. Ray E. Trussell. When Wagner completed the tour, he announced several actions he had authorized—among them establishment of a psychiatric inpatient service at Harlem Hospital.

After the Kolb committee released its report recommending decentralization of psychiatric services throughout the municipal hospital system, the Commissioner of Hospitals asked Dr. Kolb to assume responsibility for developing an inpatient psychiatric service at Harlem Hospital. Dr. Kolb agreed on the condition that he would have budgetary control. The city and Columbia University entered into a simple contract providing a lump-sum budget, thus making it possible for new staff to be recruited using university pay scales and fringe benefits.

Psychiatry was the first of the major departments at Harlem Hospital to enter into affiliation contracts with Columbia for professional staffing. The contract mandated establishment of a 40-bed inpatient psychiatric unit and supporting services. The university, for its part, contracted to provide consultation for the organization, development, and operation of a graduate training program for psychiatrists and allied professionals and to operate a hospital psychiatric service. Salaries for all professional and some administrative staff together with a small amount for emergency equipment and supplies were paid from the lump-sum budget controlled by the department's university-appointed director, with accountability to New York City's Department of Hospitals through the university's apparatus for administering affiliation contracts. Beginning July 1, 1962, the Department assumed responsibility for providing needed psychiatric services to eligible individuals residing in the Harlem Hospital district.

From this has followed an affiliation of more than 30 years between Columbia and Harlem Hospital, which has included many faculty appointments and the development of a Department of Psychiatry that was a pacesetter in using a general hospital psychiatry unit as the professional administrative hub of a system providing comprehensive psychiatric services to a defined community. The 1961 recommendations of the National Joint Commission on Mental Health provided valuable guidelines and support in planning the comprehensive services envisioned as well as justifying their budgets.

To fulfill these mandates, the basic developmental structure was laid down at the outset and function was defined. Key positions were described as to scope and responsibilities. Salaries were made sufficiently realistic to enable the department to compete for scarce professional personnel, yet were well within established norms in the various disciplines as required by university standards.

The Task

Since the average income of the 400,000 residents of the district was about one-third less than the city average, a large proportion of the population was (and still is today) eligible for municipal hospital services. In addition to problems incident to low socioeconomic status, the district's population is also beset by the psychological effects of social and economic discrimination and de facto segregation. It also suffers an extremely high incidence of psychiatric disorder. The Central Harlem Health District ranked number 1 in state hospital admissions and juvenile delinquency rates in the entire city in the 1960 census. Neighboring health districts partially included in the Harlem Hospital District occupied rank orders number 6 and 7 in state hospital admission rates and rank orders number 3 and 6 in juvenile delinquency rates, respectively.

In 1962, the Harlem Hospital Department of Psychiatry was, for all practical purposes, the only facility offering general psychiatric services other than hospitalization to adult residents of the hospital district and in addition had to provide outpatient services to many children in the area.

Early Planning

The plan was to develop, as soon as possible, a 40-bed inpatient service in space to be made available on the top (9th) floor of the "K" Building, at that time the newest of the existing Harlem Hospital buildings—only 5 years old. Ultimately, five floors of the K Building would be designated for use by the new department after completion of a new Harlem Hospital building, projected for the late 1960s. In the meantime, psychiatric outpatient services would remain where they were, on an upper floor of one of the oldest buildings in the hospital complex. Necessary structural changes on "9K," as the psychiatric inpatient service floor came to be called, would require about 1 year. The fact that the newly appointed director, Elizabeth B. Davis, M.D., had been a trainee as well as staff psychiatrist both at Harlem Hospital and in Columbia's Department of Psychiatry and was therefore familiar with the personnel of both institutions and with the Harlem Hospital physical plant undoubtedly contributed to the speed at which work could proceed. Crucial also was a high level of administrative support from both the hospital and the university.

Core personnel recruited by July 1, 1962, were all current or former Columbia Department of Psychiatry trainees and/or staff known to the director and committed to the task to be accomplished. They were Hugh F. Butts, M.D., as chief of inpatient services; Lawrence Cassard, M.D., as staff psychiatrist (inpatient); Lonnie MacDonald, M.D., as chief of community psychiatry; Hagop S. Mashikian, M.D. (part-time), as chief of emergency room and ward consultation services; Kathleen Goodin, M.S.W., as psychiatric social worker; and the author as department director and chief of the adult outpatient clinic. Of these, four were black, two were white, three were residents of Harlem, all lived in New York City, and one was both foreign-born and a foreign medical graduate.

Middle-level staff was recruited on the basis of the opportunity to participate in a new, dynamic program. Jobs were filled in accordance with clear, current needs as the basic program evolved. A program designed with staff collaboration becomes invested with much greater interest and personal involvement than one that because of statutory requirements must be presented already complete to a staff for their implementation.

The existing Harlem Hospital Mental Hygiene Clinic[1]—underfinanced and understaffed (four part-time psychiatrists, one social worker, one full-

---

1. The clinic was first established by the New York City Department of Hospitals in 1947 in response to escalating community demand that *some* psychiatric services be provided at Harlem Hospital beyond the transfer of patients to Bellevue for hospitalization.

time and one part-time psychologist, and one trained nurse)—had struggled throughout the 15 years of its existence to provide outpatient care in the community. Its staff had also been responsible for transfers from Harlem's emergency room and its general wards to the psychiatric receiving facility at Bellevue Hospital and for documenting the need for "medical suspension" of public-school students referred by the Board of Education. Both of these functions were sensitive issues in the community. Hence, outpatient services were promptly expanded to include:

- regular psychiatric consultation to hospital emergency room staff
- regular psychiatric consultation to staff of the hospital's general wards
- increased availability of adult outpatient services
- a separate outpatient service for children
- psychiatric consultation to community agencies
- a Day Hospital

Also, a 3-year general psychiatry residency training program was to be designed and approval obtained so that recruitment of residents could begin.

Implementation

Outpatient Services

Our earliest approaches to expanding outpatient services for the Harlem community were begun in 1962 by reevaluating the current treatment needs of the clinic's long-term patients, many of whom (in accordance with tradition) were on a schedule of weekly visits, with the goal of freeing up staff time for new patients. Davis (1968) reported that a first step was to eliminate waiting lists of a duration of 6 months or longer.

> Those who showed no change in status in either a positive or negative direction for the preceding three months were put on a schedule of clinic visits not exceeding one per month and for many, once every three months. Patients were assured that, should trouble arise, they were free to return before the next scheduled appointment. This technique permitted the immediate scheduling of initial interviews by at least one member of the staff for patients who had applied within the past few weeks. These patients were seen by a psychiatrist who referred them, as indicated, for social service care

and, in those rare instances when psychological testing was needed for diagnostic clarity, to the psychologist.

At a weekly conference, the staff reviewed all new patients who had been admitted during that week. Decisions were made about disposition, treatment modalities, and ancillary therapeutic measures. By utilizing this procedure, all clinic staff were made aware of the pressure for clinical services and encouraged to provide immediate and efficient contact with patients; this was a means of reducing the amount of clinic services needed for any one patient.

> The vast majority of those seeking services at the clinic were severely ill. Medication was a very important and useful modality of treatment. It often allowed patients who were essentially, and by virtue of experience, too distrustful of the services provided for the indigent population to establish a treatment relationship. Many patients showed the scars not only of psychiatric pathology, but of the severest types of social pathology. (Davis 1968)

Because of the scarcity of social agencies in the community, it was necessary for the staff to develop and operate a "do-it-yourself" clinic—that is, caseworkers established a working relationship with the welfare department and generated proposals to develop more effective methods of cooperation. We made use of the developing antipoverty program as a resource in the treatment of emotionally disturbed adolescents for whom remaining in the community was still a possibility. This was a reciprocal arrangement in that we became a resource for the antipoverty program.

As referrals increased, it was soon clearly demonstrated that there was a need for a variety of treatment modalities. With the recruitment of June Jackson Christmas, M.D., who had a great deal of experience and interest in the application of group methods to a clinical population, group therapy was introduced.

> Groups were formed at every age level and with every type of approach—supportive, insight, activity, and milieu-therapeutic. An alcoholics' group was established in the clinic. It was discovered that the prescribing of medication for patients in a group therapy setting permitted ventilation of fears and reassurance about these fears in a more effective way than could be done with many patients in individual sessions. (Davis 1968)

We found that a variety of modifications of then-standard psychiatric practice "reached" some members of the community in need of psychiatric care more effectively than did some of the more traditional methods because these innovative methods were, in fact, more useful to them. Thus, we began to conceive of "hard to accept" treatment methods rather than "hard to reach" patients.

In September 1962, Dr. Mashikian (chief of emergency room and ward consultation services) was joined by two part-time psychiatrists in response to the intense need for direct psychiatric emergency treatment. They also served in the adult clinic, thus providing needed linkage between emergency room and clinic staff and treatment.

On January 1, 1963, upon the eagerly anticipated arrival in the department of Dr. Virginia N. Wilking, a full-time child psychiatrist, the separate Division of Child Psychiatry was established. Soon thereafter, we succeeded in recruiting Dr. Margaret Morgan Lawrence to develop much-needed specific diagnostic and treatment services for the infant through early childhood population.

Since his appointment in 1962, Dr. MacDonald had been making contacts in the community to develop relationships with local resources clearly needed for optimum care of our patients in addition to providing liaison to related community agencies. He had already started a treatment program for heroin-addicted female patients on the general medical ward who had accepted medically managed detoxification during their hospitalization. This was the first inpatient treatment program for heroin addiction in pregnant patients (beyond detoxification) in any of the municipal general hospitals. It became the first methadone maintenance treatment program in any of the city hospitals.

Given the needs of the community, the steps taken to facilitate appropriate referral of individuals who came to the attention of any of the general hospital services, together with the increase in available psychiatric clinic staff and the use of innovative methods for improving both patient access and efficient use of staff, it is not surprising that the total number of adult and child outpatient psychiatry visits rose from 3,145 in 1961 to 11,004 in 1964.

Day Hospital and Inpatient Services

On September 1, 1962, the 10-patient Psychiatric Day Hospital opened, with follow-up services provided by the unit's staff upon the patient's discharge from intensive day hospital treatment. From its inception, Dr. Butts directed the Intensive Care Service of the department. In February 1963, a small (8-bed) inpatient service was initiated for selected female patients, for whom this was usually their first psychiatric admission. This system permitted treatment of at least some of the patients requiring 24-hour care and provided a model for continuity of care from inpatient through day hospital and outpatient phases of treatment, pending the opening of a larger and less selective inpatient service.

On July 1, 1963, the long-planned coeducational inpatient service was opened with 37 beds (instead of 40, as originally planned) for 24-hour patients, and a total of 13 day hospital places. Together, these comprised the Psychiatric Intensive Care Service.

On that same date, the first two residents began their psychiatric training at Harlem Hospital. (One of these, Dr. Pauline Edwards, recipient of an NIMH General Practitioner Psychiatry Training Grant, remained a member of the staff with increasing levels of responsibility for service and training until her retirement in 1983).

Evolution of the treatment programs of the Intensive Care Service continued under the direction of Dr. Butts, now also associate director of the department. Ward treatment consisted of all the usual modalities of care, including individual psychotherapy. In some cases this psychotherapy was intensive and aimed at achieving a degree of insight that permitted the patient to recognize the connection between the precipitating situation and the onset of illness, or behavior patterns that increased interpersonal or adaptive difficulties. Enormous effort was invested in orienting psychiatrically inexperienced nursing staff to the particularities of psychiatric nursing and to the principles of milieu therapy.[2] Daily ward conferences, in which staff and patients participated, were difficult initially. The majority of patients and nursing aides came from disadvantaged backgrounds and were insecure about speaking up to a professional staff. A staff discussion pertaining to observations and providing explanations of patient behavior followed each ward conference. Gradually, the nonprofessional nursing staff began to participate. Within 3 to 5 days of admission, patients were expected to participate in the recreational program, which took place in the gymnasium of a community center one block away from the hospital. Patients requiring services in other medical specialties attended the appropri-

---

2. The nursing staff was under the guidance of a very capable head nurse, Audrey Schween, who had been recruited from the then-experimental day hospital program of the Einstein Medical Center. Many years later, she went on to direct a training program for nurses throughout the Municipal Hospital System.

Development of a Department of Psychiatry in a General Hospital 33

ate clinic session accompanied by a staff member.[3] An active occupational therapy program provided many accessories for the dayrooms used by all patients.[4]

The same basic pattern was followed in both the day hospital and the inpatient units. Each, however, had a separate staff and separate conference and activity schedules. In July 1965, the two services were integrated, for clinical as well as administrative reasons. Dr. Butts reported that in addition to the obvious economic disadvantage of completely separate facilities, the inpatient group had come to perceive itself, as had some staff members, as having inferior status. Because the 24-hour patients were likely to be the most recently admitted, and were often still acutely disturbed and in need of close supervision, they could not attend as much of the activity therapy program as could the day hospital patients. Necessary restrictions were often perceived as suggestive of the lower status they tended to equate with "commitment," although most patients had in fact requested admission voluntarily.

Similarly, the 24-hour patients wished to have "peer relations" with day hospital patients who had an aura of "less disturbed" in their own eyes and those of visitors and relatives. In addition, they envied the patients with more privileges the opportunity to participate in more off-ward activities. From the staff's point of view, contact with patients farther advanced in their treatment was helpful in inducing attitudes of hope and greater willingness to participate fully in available therapeutic programs, and was therefore seen as "positive." In the interest of providing continuity of care, former patients were readmitted to the service whenever rehospitalization was indicated and a bed could be made available.

Aftercare for inpatients was a serious problem. Transfer from the comprehensive therapeutic approach of the ward to the diluted treatment of the clinic proved difficult for many patients. An effort was made to bridge the gap through the establishment of an "ex-patient club" that met once a week on the ward, with the regular head nurse as leader, and offered refreshments. This helped somewhat, but finally the ward staff set up its own aftercare clinic on the ward (Butts 1964, 1967).

Staff quickly became overloaded, however, in the attempt to maintain high-quality intensive care for inpatient and day hospital patients while attending to the needs of ever-increasing numbers of patients discharged

---

3. General medical and surgical clinics were also located in the K Building.
4. The activity therapy program for intensive care patients began under the supervision of Barbara Verdell, a trained and experienced occupational therapist recruited from the staff of the Einstein Day Hospital.

from intensive care for whom the "right time" for transfer to the outpatient clinic never seemed to arrive.

In addition, the residents' training program was threatened by conflicts between patient care responsibilities involved in the program and its formal teaching schedule, some of whose sessions were provided at the Columbia-Presbyterian Medical Center, a 15-minute shuttle bus ride from Harlem Hospital (Butts and Lindo 1968).

Because of an overall shortage of municipal hospital psychiatric beds in late 1967, average lengths of inpatient stays on this unit were sharply reduced (28 days in 1967 to 16 days in 1968) after implementation of a city-wide administrative policy limiting the maximum length of stay.[5] This change sharply aggravated the organizational problems previously described and was a factor in alerting staff to the need to develop more long-term effective approaches to chronic mental illness (Davis et al. 1968).

Rehabilitation

During this period—the early to mid-1960s—the New York State Department of Mental Hygiene's deinstitutionalization program was getting into full swing, and many of the state's aftercare patients found their way to our department's outpatient services via referral from the emergency room or the ward consultation service, or self-referral to our adult outpatient clinic.

The group therapy program, under Dr. Christmas's leadership, expanded to meet this need by instituting an outpatient activity therapy program. At first the program used a socialization therapy format in which participants read and discussed newspapers over coffee; it gradually evolved to include a combined occupational/recreational therapy program offered to outpatients one to three times weekly, according to their need. It was staffed by an experienced occupational therapist, Delores Chandler, who was assisted by a gifted paraprofessional, Frances Brock-Davies, selected for her previous experience in organizing community cultural programs (Christmas and Davis 1965).

With this additional component of outpatient clinic service, inpatient staff felt more secure in referring patients discharged from intensive care.

---

5. The maximum stay limit was first decreased to 21 days. This proved unfeasible and was later raised to 35 days.

Active liaison and cooperation with the adult clinic, now headed by Dr. Jean Keller, rapidly developed to provide continuity of care through related and *communicating* staff.

As a result of the more positive outcome for many of the very chronic patients in this program, as well as in response to pressures on the intensive care services, we faced the necessity for providing specifically rehabilitative services for deinstitutionalized patients. For many of these, the prospect at that time was years of isolated existence broken only by monthly visits to the clinic to replenish the medication that permitted them to remain outside the hospital. But that kind of aftercare program did little to give such individuals the means for living *in* the world rather than at the edge of it, as Dr. MacDonald had demonstrated in a study of posthospital patients (Fisch and MacDonald 1964).

With Dr. Christmas as principal investigator, a federally financed research grant was obtained to develop and evaluate a program of psychosocial and vocational rehabilitation for posthospital patients with chronic mental illness. The New York City Commissioner of Hospitals and Commissioner of Mental Health strongly supported this effort. The Department of Hospitals funded acquisition of the necessary quarters in a newly renovated loft building a few blocks away from the hospital. Ten years later, in 1977, this program, by then institutionalized as one of the department's continuing services and under the direction of Gladys Egri, M.D. (Dr. Christmas having moved on to become New York City Commissioner of Mental Health), was awarded the APA's Certificate of Significant Achievement (Christmas 1966, 1972a, 1972b; Daniels 1968).

Social Services

In contrast to other affiliated and unaffiliated departments of the hospital, social work in the Department of Psychiatry was from the beginning included under the affiliation contract as an allied profession, and social workers were fully integrated into the administrative as well as clinical work of the department.

Early in 1964, Maurice V. Russell, M.S.W., Ed.D, was recruited to direct psychiatric social work throughout the department. By July of that year, the psychiatric social work staff had grown to nine full-time and two part-time master's-level social workers—as many as were available to all the other hospital services combined.

Training

Since the major commitment of the university under the affiliation agreement was to provide, through its Harlem affiliation staff, a training program for psychiatrists and allied professionals, attention given to training was early, close, and persistent.

In 1962–1963, two PGY 4 (3rd-year) residents transferred from other programs and two PGY 2 (1st-year) residents were accepted to begin training July 11, 1963. The 3-year residency program in general psychiatry, with the author as director of training, had already been formulated and conditionally approved.

An 8-week seminar on psychiatric aspects of nursing for registered nurses was offered during May and June 1963 as part of the effort to recruit nurses to staff the 37-bed coeducational inpatient service scheduled to open July 1, 1963.

From the beginning, training of psychiatric residents and other therapy staff was enriched by supervision of their psychodynamically oriented psychotherapy by Raymond Raskin, M.D., and Victor Goldin, M.D., both graduates of Columbia's Psychoanalytic Clinic for Research and Training, and of their group therapy by June Jackson Christmas, M.D., a psychoanalytically trained group therapist.

Psychiatric Residency Training

The essence of the department's approach to residency training (by then fully approved) throughout the tenure of its first director (1962–1978) was outlined in its 1965 brochure, *Training in Psychiatry—Harlem Hospital Center*.

- The resident should learn how to relate an increasing knowledge of psychodynamics to an increasing clinical knowledge of psychiatric disorders.
- Learning in these areas must be integrated with the knowledge of basic biological sciences, pathophysiology, organic pathology and clinical medicine, to which must be added
- A special familiarity with neurophysiology, neurochemistry, neuropathology, and neurology.
- Disturbance in functioning can be understood by the resident's viewing the individual as a psychobiologic unit continuously interacting with his own particular physical and social milieu.

- The resident learns about various frames of reference through their exposition in guided reading, lectures, seminars, as well as through interaction with the staff (of all disciplines) in conferences and supervision.
- This philosophy of training is implemented through a coordinated teaching program, which makes maximum use of the available clinical facilities.

In 1965, our commitment to psychiatric training was further reinforced with the establishment of an approved child psychiatry residency training program, with Dr. Virginia N. Wilking as director. Recruitment of trainees for both the adult and the child psychiatry residency programs was both slow and difficult. But by July 1, 1969, 6 of our 14 approved residency slots were filled, and by the following July all were filled. Half our residents in 1969 were graduates of American medical schools, primarily Howard and Meharry. This was a long-hoped-for development, to which the Civil Rights Movement and student protests of the early 1960s had made a significant contribution by opening up far wider opportunities throughout the nation for black physicians to obtain specialty training.

Meanwhile, in response to requests from the New York state hospitals serving New York City (Manhattan and Rockland Psychiatric Centers) to assist their residents by providing training in general hospital psychiatry, specifically emergency room and ward consultation experience (as they provided 2 months of state hospital experience for our residents), Harlem Hospital designed a 3-month rotation for 3d-year state hospital residents on these services. These rotations proved very successful with the state hospital residents.

The 1970 appointment of Bruce L. Ballard, M.D., to an NIMH Career Psychiatry Teacher Training Program Fellowship at Harlem was enormously important in the implementation and development of the new residency training program as well as in providing a readily available mentor for the residents. Until that time, responsibility for general residents' training had rested on the shoulders of the increasingly busy senior staff, with the author as training director. Upon completion of his fellowship, Dr. Ballard was appointed residency training director and continued in that role until 1976, when he was succeeded by Dr. I. Jay Averbach.

Training for Allied Professionals

Early in 1964, shortly after Dr. Russell joined us, plans got under way to place a Columbia University School of Social Work student unit in the Department of Psychiatry. These plans were implemented in the fall of 1964, and the department continued assigning Columbia social work students to placements at Harlem during the appointments of both Mrs. Edna Ford, Dr. Russell's successor as associate director of social services (psychiatry), and her successor, Kenneth Erskine, M.S.W. A number of graduates of the school who trained at Harlem later returned as staff members. Some of them have gone on to make noteworthy contributions in their field.

Until the 1970s, training for psychologists was limited to group placements of 1st-year doctoral candidates in the clinical psychiatry program at Teachers College, Columbia University. The clinical assignments were primarily observational, involving observing the function of a psychiatric service and following the course of a particular patient's treatment on the service. After the appointment of Carol Garmiza, Ph.D., as the department's chief psychologist, a clinical psychology internship program was initiated. Its participants were highly valued members of the therapeutic team, especially in child and adolescent psychiatry.

From the beginning, training for the nursing staff was integrated with clinical programs throughout the department, but from time to time opportunities for psychiatric nursing experience and training were requested by and made available to Harlem Hospital's and Columbia University's schools of nursing for both pre- and post-R.N. training. Residents of Columbia's training program in occupational therapy were also provided placement in our activity therapy programs after their rapid evolution in the late 1960s.

Training of mental health paraprofessionals was conducted primarily on the intensive care service, as described earlier, and on the Rehabilitation Service, where the potential of undereducated and underemployed community residents to perform such work had been effectively demonstrated (Christmas 1966, 1972b).

Interdepartmental Relationships

As the psychiatric service was being developed, other newly affiliated services in the hospital were also expanding. In 1963, the new chief of obstetrics and gynecology had established an effective family-planning clinic. Prenatal care became more individualized, and opportunity was provided for more collaboration with our OB/GYN colleagues. For instance, interest in jointly providing better services for our many unwed teenage mothers resulted in a program in our Division of Child Psychiatry that combined casework and group therapy for very young women having a first baby. The intention of the program was to help these young mothers reenter the stream of educational and vocational life after their babies were born and to prevent the vicious cycle of unwed motherhood, rejection, isolation, and repeated pregnancy.

Inevitable compromises regarding allocation of existing space and equipment had to be negotiated within the hospital "family." It is not surprising that bureaucratic as well as professional ambivalence toward psychiatry as a discipline found expression through administrative maneuvers as well as in clinical matters.

After July 1964, with the staff expanded to include residents assigned to rotations on the consultation service and, for the first time, a full-time psychiatrist, Austin Moore, M.D. (who joined us from Downstate Medical Center in Brooklyn as chief of the ward consultation service), it was possible to add direct treatment for patients on medical and surgical services to the diagnostic and consultative services previously provided. Observation by medical and surgical staff of the results of numerous examples of effective psychiatric treatment for their patients had a salutary effect on relations between the psychiatry department and the staff of other hospital departments. The elective offered in psychiatry became used more frequently and effectively by interns and residents in the hospital's other training programs.

Stocktaking—the 5th Year

During the 5 years after the department was established, the various points of view and competencies of its staff were welded into a working force that by 1967 was providing five core services:

- 24-hour, 7 days/week psychiatric emergency services in the hospital's emergency room
- psychiatric inpatient and transitional day hospital services, averaging 400 admissions per year
- sophisticated outpatient clinic and day treatment (defined as three to five sessions weekly of between 2 and 5 hours in length) for large annual caseloads of adults and children
- Consultation to all other clinical services of the hospital, with collaborative treatment as indicated, for a total of 5,890 visits in that year
- Highly organized psychosocial and vocational rehabilitation services for individuals with chronic mental illness

Community Psychiatry

Although no specific contractual obligation to develop a community psychiatry service had been in the original commitment to establish an inpatient psychiatric unit with supporting services, the inclinations and training of our staff along with the complex intertwining of social and psychiatric problems in the population we served permitted us to address directly some of the underlying mental health problems of the community.

Several senior staff members who were trained psychoanalysts viewed much of the presenting psychopathology as causally related to the widespread existence of emotional and social deprivation and saw these as major contributing factors to the development of clinical psychosis, neurosis, and personality disorder. The contribution of a strong division of child psychiatry to this developmental view cannot be overestimated. The inclusion of trained community psychiatrists on the senior staff greatly enhanced our awareness of epidemiologic and public mental health approaches to the clinical problems faced.

The contribution of Columbia University's Department of Psychiatry in the development of the Harlem program had begun long before the affiliation was established. Acceptance of black physicians for psychiatric and psychoanalytic training as well as for training in community psychiatry at Columbia had preceded by many years the university's decision to affiliate with Harlem. The acceptance of Margaret Morgan Lawrence, M.D., as its first black psychiatry resident (in the late 1960s) had been greatly facilitated by strategically timed interventions of one particular Columbia faculty member, Viola W. Bernard, M.D. A psychoanalyst and lifelong instigator of and campaigner for equal opportunities for psychiatric training at all levels for members of minority groups, particularly blacks, she was also the first director of Columbia's Division of Community Psychiatry. This training program was based jointly in the university's Department of Psychiatry and its School of Public Health.

In addition to and complementing the perceptions of psychiatric staff, a competent, professional social work staff pointed up the great need for and abysmal lack of basic social services in our community. Some of the Harlem community's sociopsychiatric needs were defined for staff in their discussions at various conferences and also during visits and consultations to community agencies and personnel. These opportunities for communication were sought by both the community and the staff. Out of these discussions came several specific programs, some of which represented joint efforts to ameliorate community-recognized problems.

A daily recreational group therapy program that was developed for emotionally disturbed boys is one example of these programs. Several agencies, including an antipoverty program and the Domestic Peace Corps, contributed to the effort. This program evolved into the Harlem Child Study Center, a full-fledged daily therapeutic educational and recreational program recognized by the New York City Board of Education as a special school, with its own public school number and a principal and teaching staff provided by that board. The recreation groups, integrated with the school program, continued as a major therapeutic tool under the knowledgeable supervision of a particularly talented member of the original Domestic Peace Corps group. A very active parent contact and parent group therapy component was conducted by trained social workers on our staff. This comprehensive program regularly achieved its goal of successfully returning boys to their local public schools after 1 to 2 years of attendance.

In response to passage of the Community Mental Health Act of 1963, and with support by all appropriate administrative bodies—state, city, and university—a CMHC grant application was developed that would have provided child and adolescent inpatient services in the K Building and new, improved facilities for psychiatric outpatients on a projected new Harlem Hospital Ambulatory Care Center.

Administration

Clearly, all the activities described in this chapter could not have been instituted or carried on without a devoted administrative staff. The position of affiliation coordinator was created in 1963 and was filled, with skill and devotion, for the succeeding 20 years by Ernest Wilderson.

Essential to efficient administration of the department was the appointment, after several predecessors, of Rosalie Landy as secretary to the department's director. (Landy is now executive director of the New York County District Branch of the American Psychiatric Association.)

By 1966, with a total professional staff of 56, 28 of whom were psychiatrists; a considerable budget; and planning under way for a projected community mental health center, it seemed wise to obtain the services of a trained hospital administrator, as was being done in other affiliated departments. Hence, Richard Perry, M.S., a graduate of the Columbia University School of Public Health's training program in hospital administration, joined the staff as its first departmental administrator.

By December 1968 the new general hospital building was nearly completed, and the vacating of four upper floors of the K Building was imminent. By this time it had become apparent that the city was not yet prepared to proceed with the projected Ambulatory-CMHC Building at Harlem Hospital Center, and plans had been made for modest renovation of that space originally allocated for psychiatry's use for expanded inpatient, day hospital and day treatment programs for children, and some outpatient services. In addition, a separate area for psychiatric emergency services was provided, and the off-site rehabilitation/child psychiatry facility was retained.

In 1968, Sheldon Zimberg, M.D., M.P.H., who had succeeded Dr. MacDonald as chief of community psychiatry, obtained a grant from the New York State Department of Mental Hygiene to study ambulatory alcohol detoxification. The alcoholism treatment program that emerged was housed in the neighboring New York City Public Health Center. Experience in this program demonstrated the need to provide within the Harlem community 24-hour, medically controlled alcohol detoxification (Zimberg 1974). Efforts were initiated that, a few years later, were rewarded by establishment of an appropriately designed and furnished detox unit in newly available space in the K Building. In 1972 community alcoholism treatment services were expanded and relocated to more spacious quarters in a medical office building in the community.

Also noted by Dr. Zimberg and his staff, and then systematically surveyed, were the psychiatric needs of the community's geriatric population. They learned that disproportionately small numbers of over-65 individuals were referred to the adult clinic. Because they were presenting in the general hospital emergency room, they were all too frequently—and often unnecessarily—transferred to the local state hospital. As a result, a specialized geriatric psychiatry daily outpatient program was established (Zimberg 1968).

Consolidation

The relocation of previously scattered services into the K Building during 1969 finally afforded a breathing period for consolidation, integration, and institutionalization. By January 1, 1969, the department staff totaled 150, including all affiliation professionals (40 of whom were full- or part-time psychiatrists).

Inevitable changes were in the making, however. Dr. Hugh Butts, chief of intensive care services and associate director of the department since 1962, announced his plan to accept an appointment as director of the

Bronx Psychiatric Center. Fortunately no lapse in leadership occurred, as Jack Sheps, M.D., a respected and experienced senior colleague, was promptly recruited to succeed Dr. Butts. Expansion of adult ambulatory care services had benefited greatly over the years from the leadership of Dr. Austin Moore, through his teaching role in all of the outpatient services as well as in his original bailiwick, the Ward Consultation Service. In 1970 he was appointed departmental associate director for ambulatory care. His responsibilities now included the adult clinic, the emergency room, and the consultation service, each of which was headed by a chief psychiatrist. Those who filled these and other positions over the succeeding years included Drs. Peter Schween, Gideon Nachumi, and Emery Hetrick.

Child psychiatry senior staff were also greatly augmented during this period. After completing child psychiatry training, Dr. Carol Leal, an early general psychiatry resident at Harlem, returned to staff as a full-time assistant to Dr. Wilking. Other former residents, Esther Roberts, M.D. (with a Columbia M.P.H. in community psychiatry), and Raymond Ransom, M.D., had also rejoined the staff—in community psychiatry and alcoholism services, respectively.

Dr. Zimberg, now responsible for a large alcoholism treatment service, was succeeded as chief of community psychiatry by another Columbia Division of Community Psychiatry graduate, John Rosenberger, M.D., M.P.H.

The psychiatry residency training program, with Dr. Bruce Ballard now training director, filled all its slots from a progressively larger applicant pool of both American and foreign medical graduates. The selection process was a team effort, and great care was taken to choose well-qualified individuals who would be able to obtain maximum benefit from the training program and to contribute effectively to meeting the service needs of the department and the community.

Increases in the department's budgets necessitated by its expansion of services were provided under three different mayoral administrations. Throughout the period the city viewed the budgets as productive in terms of volume of clinical services provided and cost-effective in terms of clinical outcomes, as documented by clinical research and evaluative studies (Davis et al. 1984).

By July 1, 1970, physical renovations in the K Building had been completed except for those necessary for the planned child and adolescent inpatient services. However, day treatment programs for children occupied the space intended for these (on floors 5K and 7K) on a "swing," that is, temporary basis.

During the late 1970s, New York City's infamous financial crisis brought strict budgetary limitations for city services and prevented implementation of the department's plans to establish child and adolescent inpatient services.

The inauguration of a new state psychiatric center for children on neighboring Ward's Island (in the East River, off 125th Street) also eased the pressure to provide these services in the Harlem district. The department, however, continued addressing the problems whose solutions were being delayed.

Professional staff throughout this period remained relatively stable, with only one change at senior levels. After the premature death in 1976 of Dr. Sheps, who had in 1970 shepherded the department as it withstood a 2-month-long "sit-in" by a local community group opposed to the expansion of psychiatric services, Dr. Seymour Gers, previously chief of the psychiatric inpatient service at the Downstate Medical Center's teaching hospital in Brooklyn, New York, assumed the duties of associate director and chief of intensive care services.

While developing inpatient, emergency, general, consultation/treatment, rehabilitation, and addiction services as well as training programs in general and child psychiatry and psychiatric components of training for allied professionals, the department had both the need and the opportunity to explore and refine the day treatment modality. Multifaceted day treatment programs for each age group from early childhood through old age were established. We found this modality of treatment to be a very flexible and cost-effective method of addressing the specific clinical needs shared by defined groups of patients. It was our experience that if appropriate emphasis is given to the parameters of age, diagnosis, and prescribed focus of therapeutic effort, attendance at such programs is greatly enhanced, and thus the programs' vulnerability to budget cuts is markedly reduced. (As an example, for the year 1976, the department's service activities report listed 11 separate day treatment programs, with a total of 43,023 visits to these programs).

The strong potential of day treatment for strengthening existing family and community support systems extends therapeutic gains made during treatment as well as the clinical gains made through more traditional methods of treatment with which it often forms part of a therapeutic continuum.

Thus, by 1977 a far-reaching and innovative program of psychiatric services to the Harlem community had been firmly established and was professionally recognized (Davis 1974). Our mandates had been fulfilled and our basic goals achieved.

References

Butts HF: The organization of a psychiatric day hospital. J Nat Med Assoc 56:381–389, 1964

Butts HF: The Harlem Hospital Center Psychiatric Day Hospital—A three-year evaluation. J Nat Med Assoc 59:273–277, 1967

Butts HF, Lindo T: Continuity of care on an intensive psychiatric treatment unit. A two year evaluation. J Nat Med Assoc 60(5): 408–414, 1968

Christmas JJ: Group methods in training and practice: non-professional mental health personnel in a deprived community. Am J Orthopsychiatry 36(3): 410–419, 1966

Christmas JJ: Group rehabilitative approaches in socially and economically deprived communities. In Progress in Group and Family Therapy. Edited by Sager CJ, Kaplan S. New York, Brunner/Mazel, 764–773, 1972a

Christmas JJ: Philosophy and practice of socio-psychiatric rehabilitation in economically deprived communities. In Progress in Community Mental Health. Edited by Bellack L, Barten H. New York, Grune, 1972b

Christmas JJ, Davis EB: Group therapy program with the socially deprived in community psychiatry. Int J Group Psychother 15:464–467, 1965

Daniels MS: Social and Community Service Annual for Division of Rehabilitation Services, Dept. of Psychiatry, Harlem Hospital Center. September 1968

Davis EB: The clinical practice of community psychiatry at Harlem Hospital. J Hillside Hospital 17(1):8–12, 1968

Davis EB, Butts HF, Lindo T: Some implications of time-limited general hospital psychiatric inpatient treatment for outcome of hospitalization. Community Mental Health J 8(2):92–101, 1972

Davis EB: Ghetto psychiatry: Harlem version. Psychiatric Annals 4(4,5):6–59, 7–83, April, May, 1974

Davis EB, Egri G, Caton C: Outcomes of care systems for chronic patients. J Nat Med Assoc 76(1):67–73, 1984

Fisch M, MacDonald L: Community-centered treatment of schizophrenia. Am J Orthopsychiatry 34(7):652–658

The 1977 APA Achievement Award winners: Hosp and Comm Psych 29(11): 524–550, 1977

Trussell RE: Symposium on the Hospitals of New York City. Bull New York Acad Med 37:524–550, 1961

Trussell RE: The municipal hospital system in transition. Bull New York Acad Med 38(4), April 1962

Zimberg S: Outpatient geriatric psychiatry in an urban ghetto with non-professional workers. Paper presented at the annual meeting of the American Psychiatric Association, May 1968

Zimberg S: Evaluation of alcoholism treatment in Harlem. Q J Studies on Alcohol 35:550–557, June 1974

Early Pioneers
in Black Psychiatry

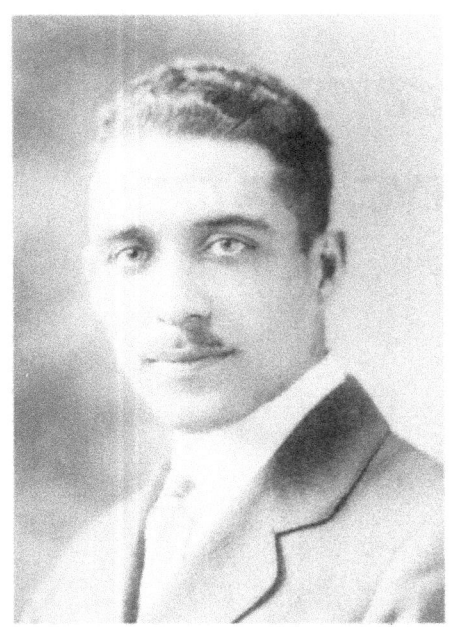

Walter Adams, M.D.

Prince Barker, M.D.

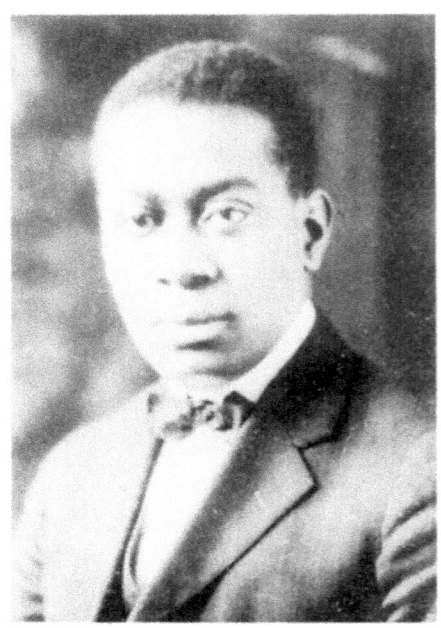

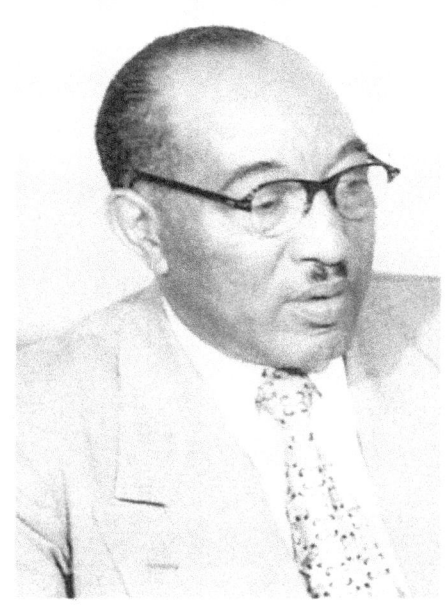

George Branch, M.D.

Herbert Erwin, M.D.
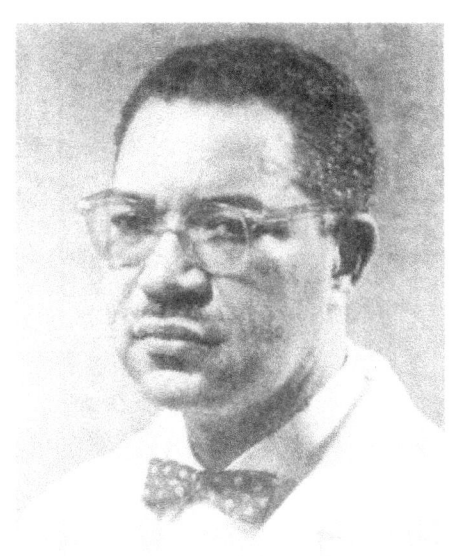

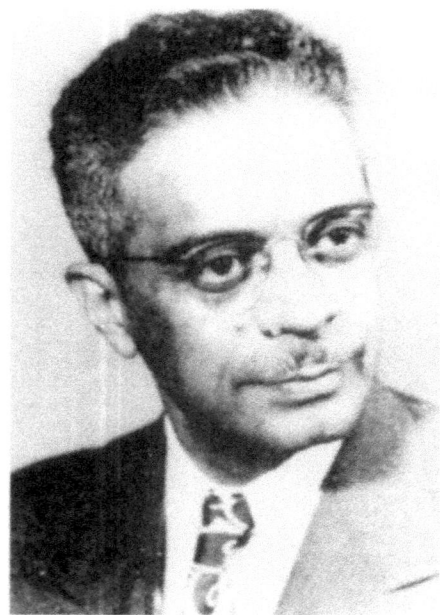

Raphael Hernandez, M.D.

Charles Prudhomme, M.D.

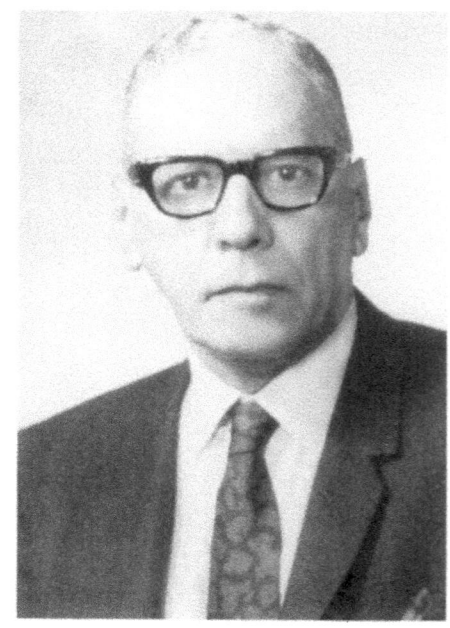

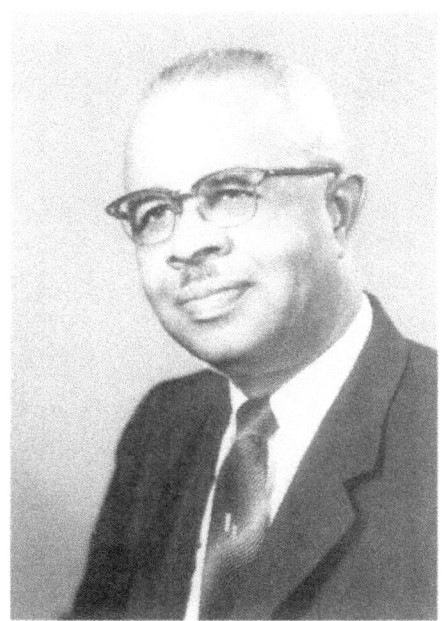

Toussaint Tilden, M.D.

Ernest Y. Williams, M.D.

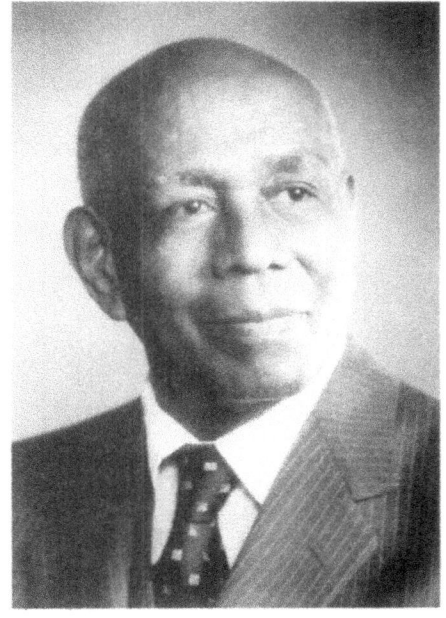

Volume Contributors

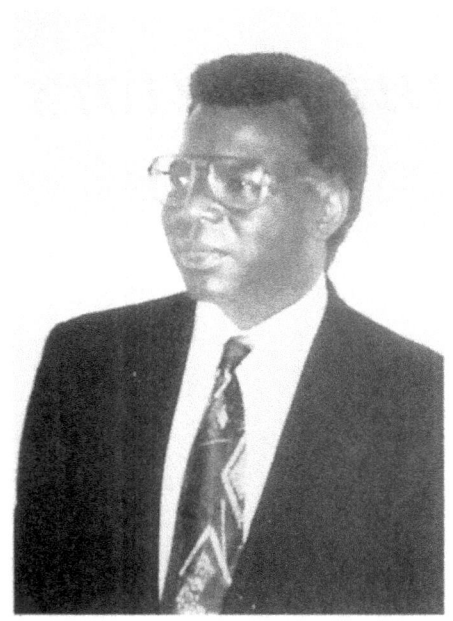

Victor R. Adebimpe, M.D.

F. M. Baker, M.D., M.P.H.

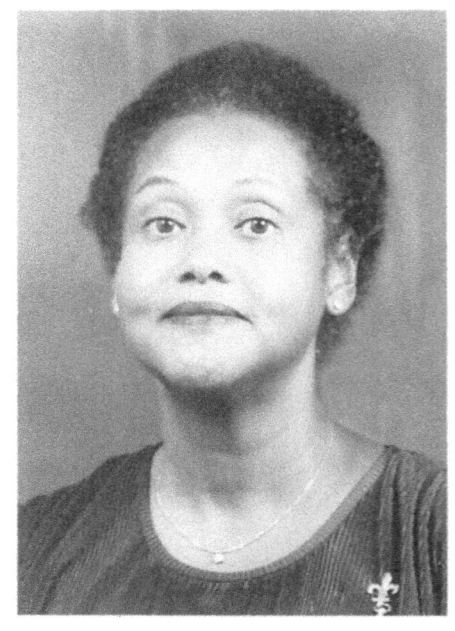

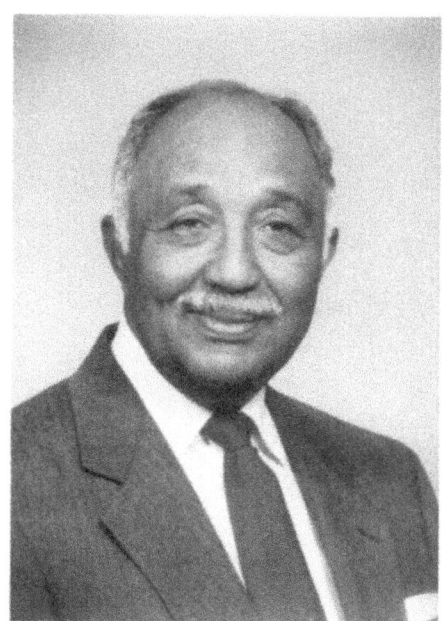

James E. Baker, M.D.

Bruce L. Ballard, M.D.

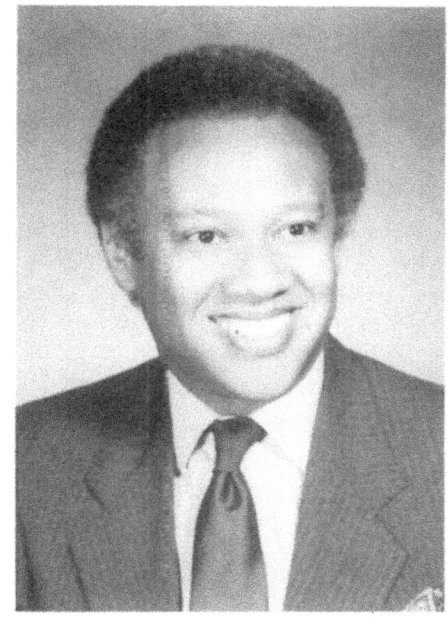

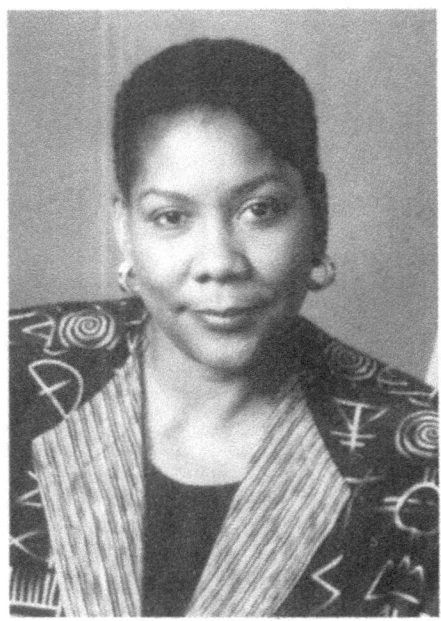

Irma J. Bland, M.D.

Clotilde Dent Bowen,
M.D., F.A.P.M., (L.)APA

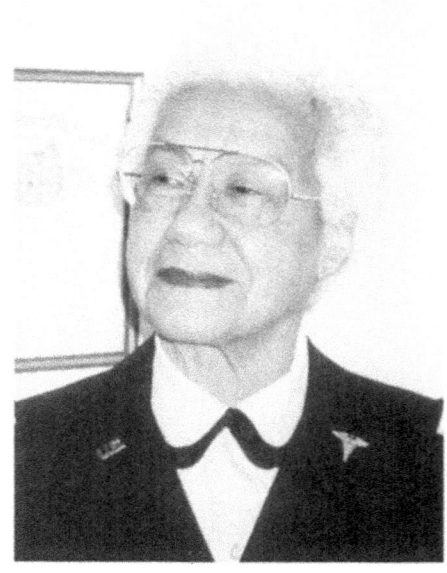

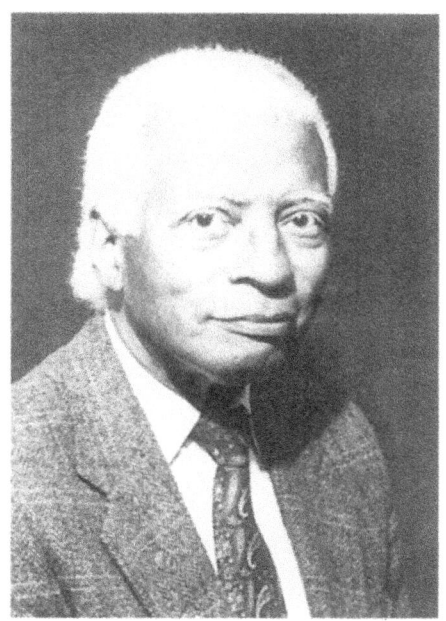

Hugh F. Butts, M.D.

Joshua W. Calhoun, M.D.

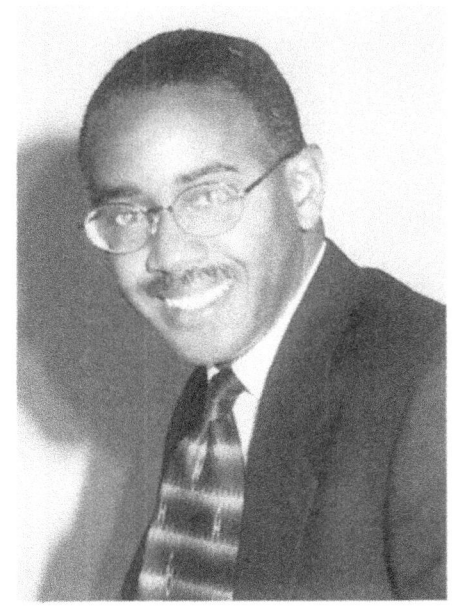

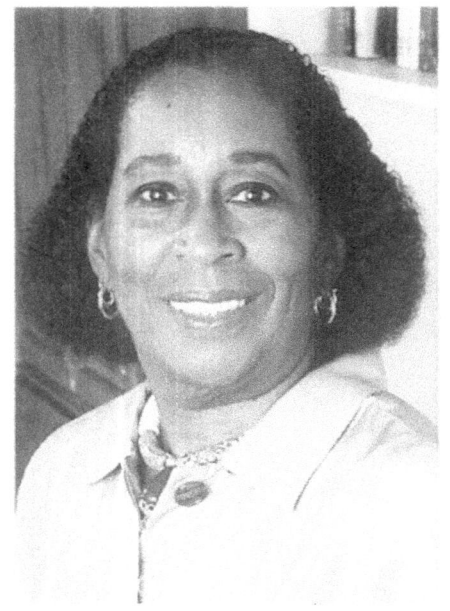

June Jackson Christmas, M.D.

James L. Collins Sr.,
M.D., F.A.P.A.

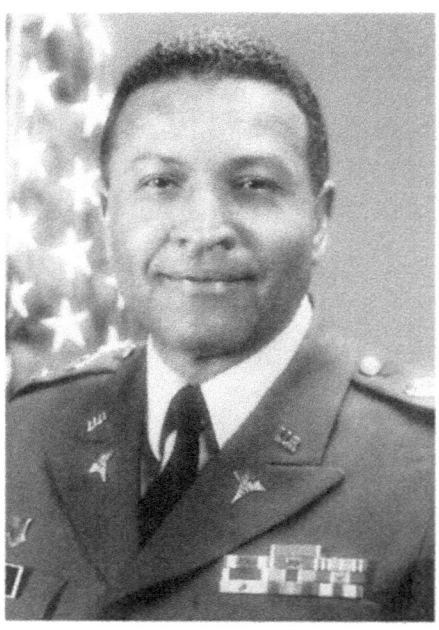

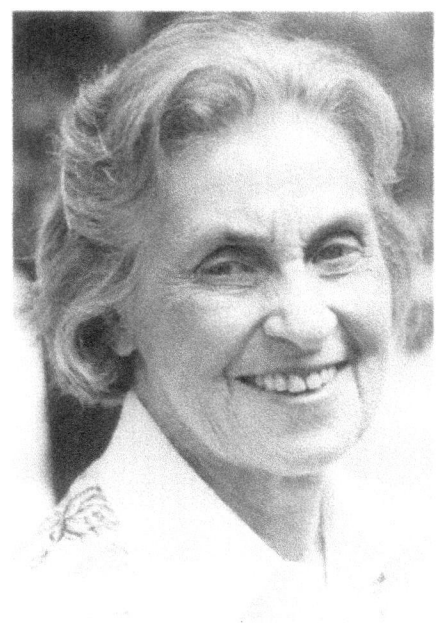

Elizabeth B. Davis, M.D.

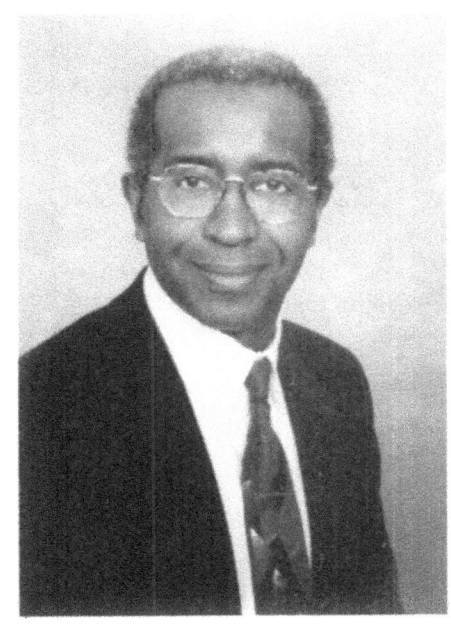

Henry E. Edwards, M.D.

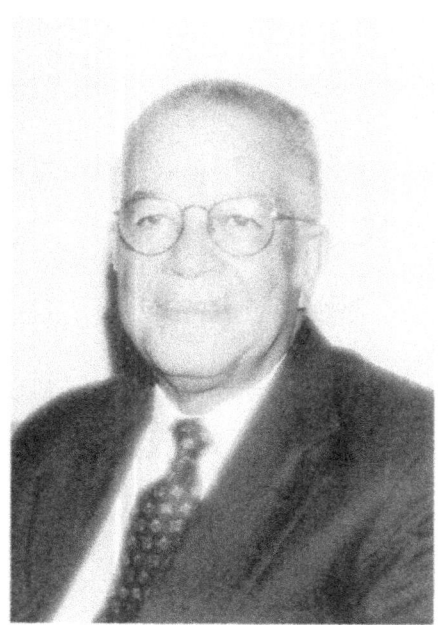

Lloyd C. Elam, M.D.

John Hope Franklin, Ph.D.

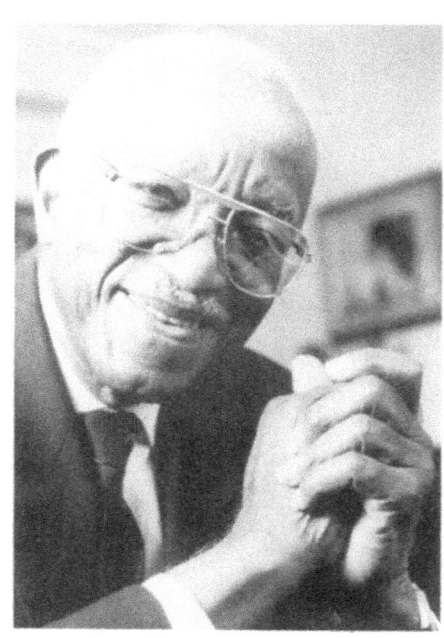

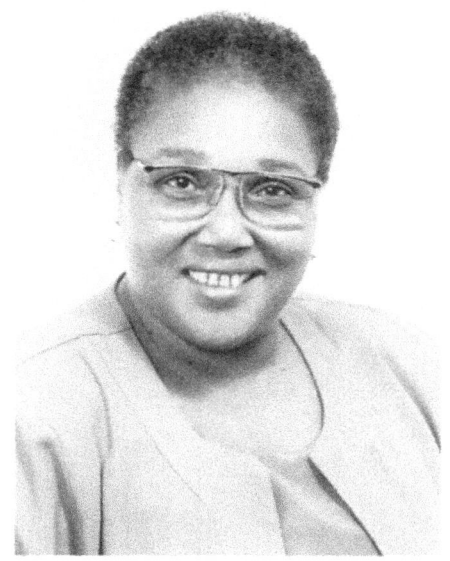

Ruth L. Fuller, M.D.

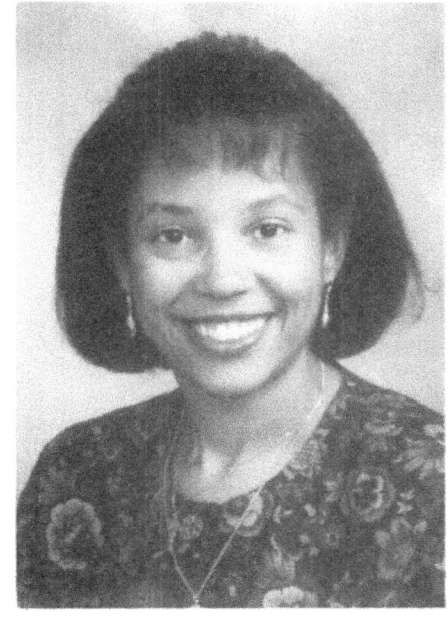

Tana A. Grady-Weliky, M.D.

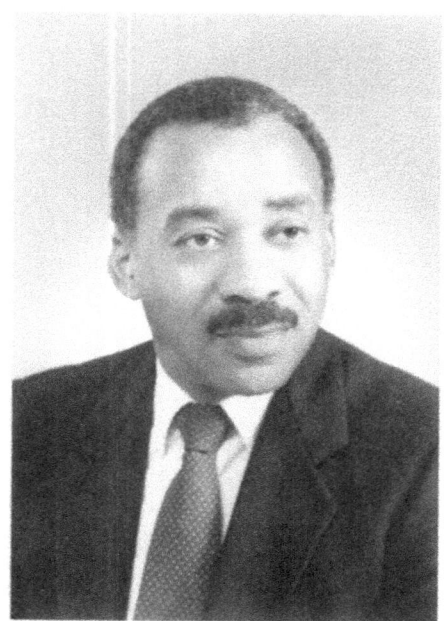

Billy E. Jones, M.D., M.S.

Ledro R. Justice, M.D.

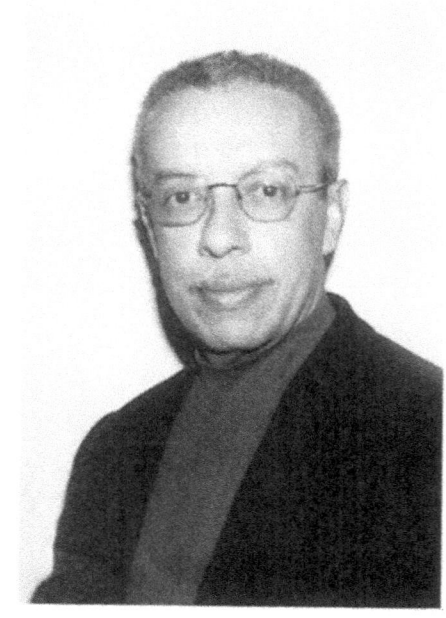

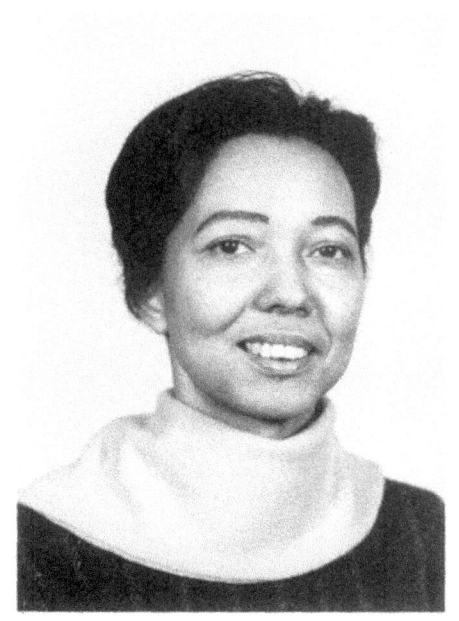

Mildred Mitchell-Bateman, M.D.

Donna M. Norris, M.D.

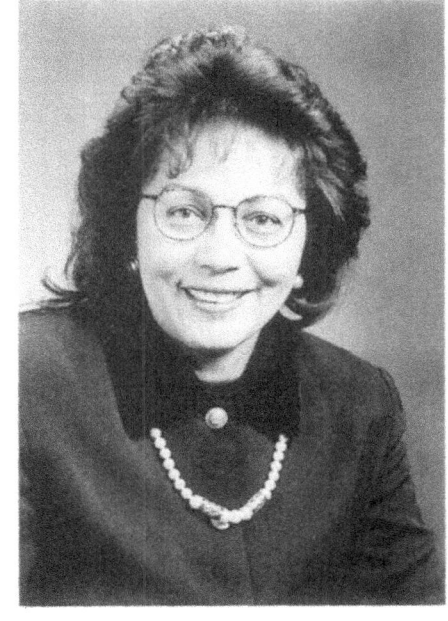

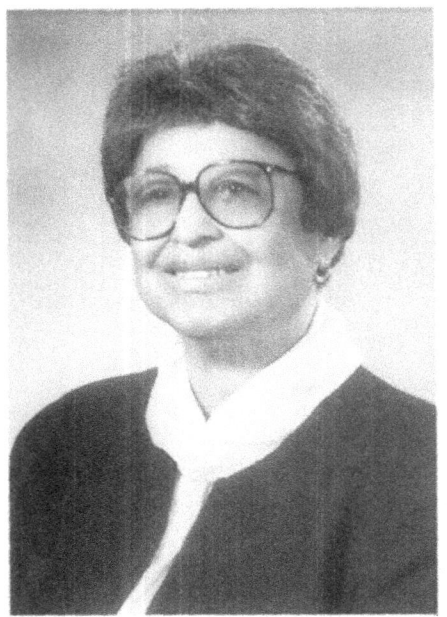

Jeanne Spurlock, M.D.

Harry H. Wright, M.D., M.B.A.

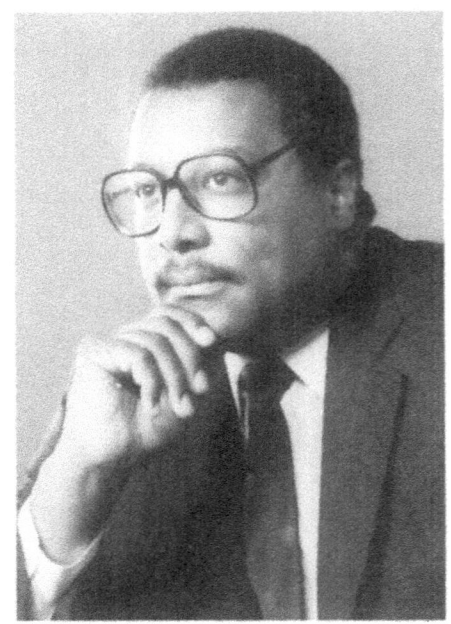

Hospitals

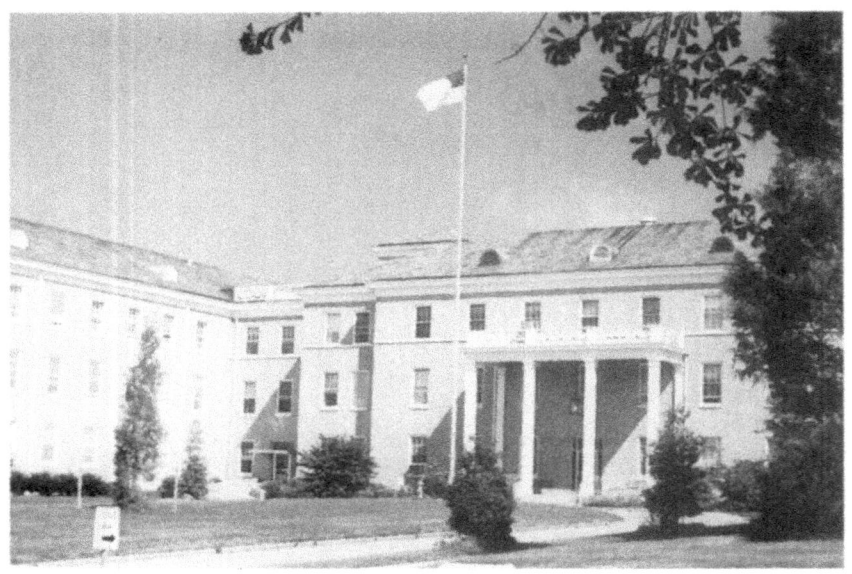

Tuskegee Veterans Administration (VA) Hospital, Tuskegee, Alabama

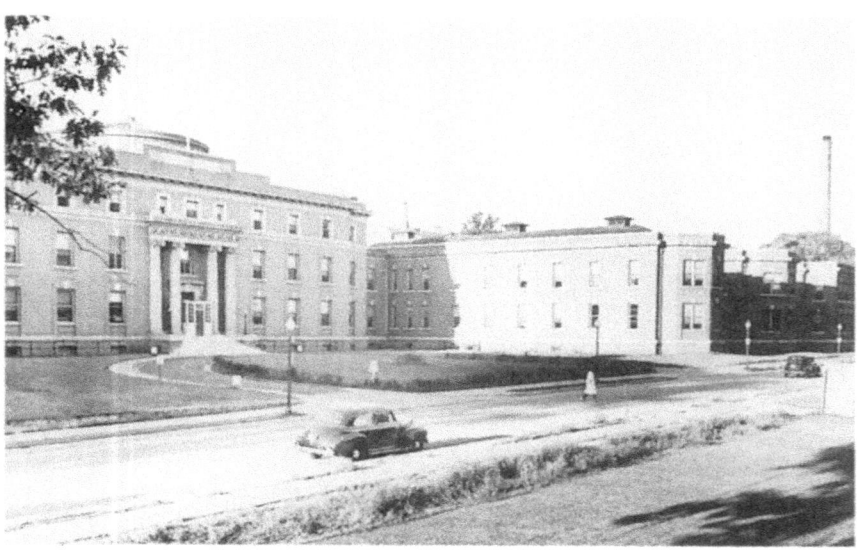

Freedmen's Hospital of Howard University College of Medicine, Washington, DC

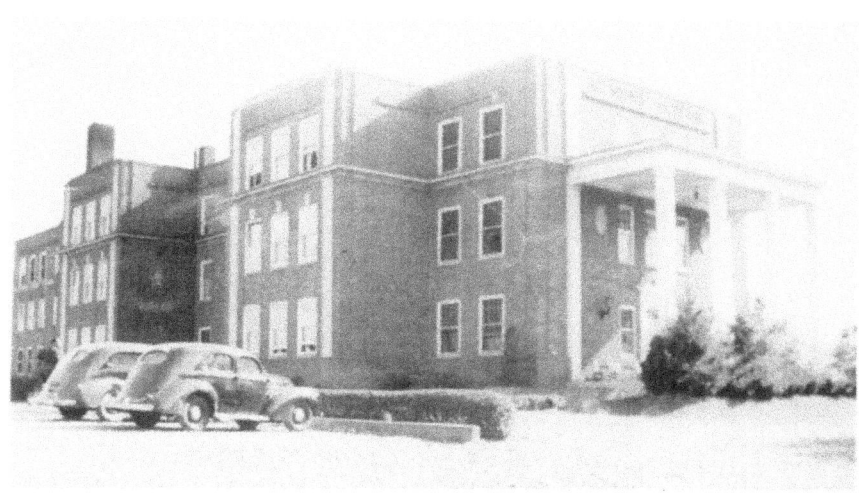

Lakin State Hospital, Lakin, West Virginia

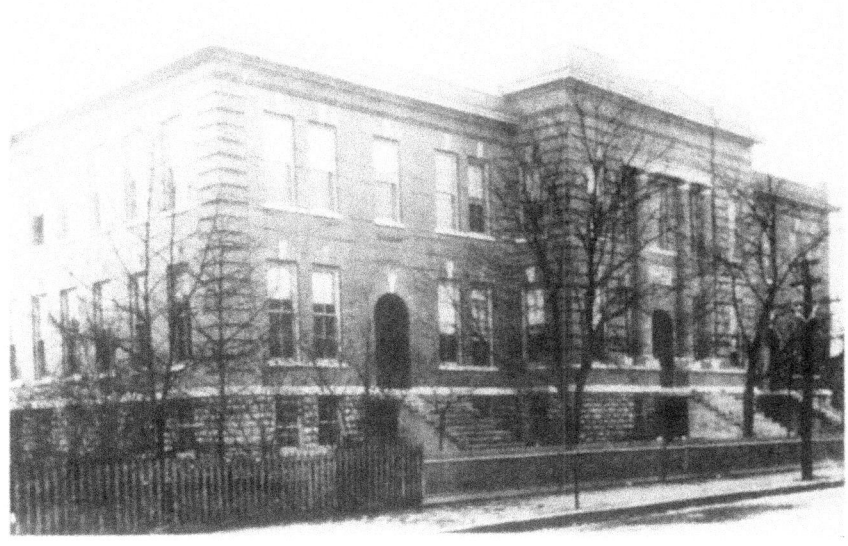

George W. Hubbard Hospital of Meharry Medical College, Nashville, Tennessee

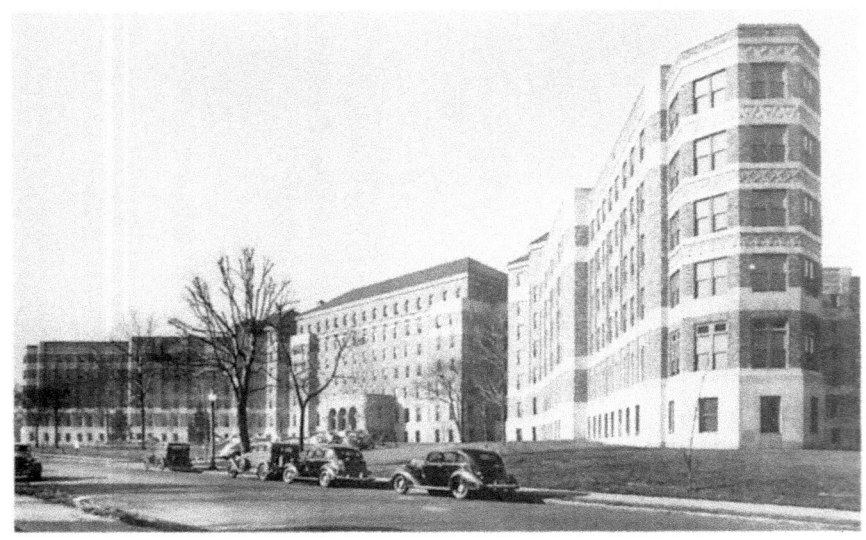

Homer G. Phillips Hospital, St. Louis, Missouri

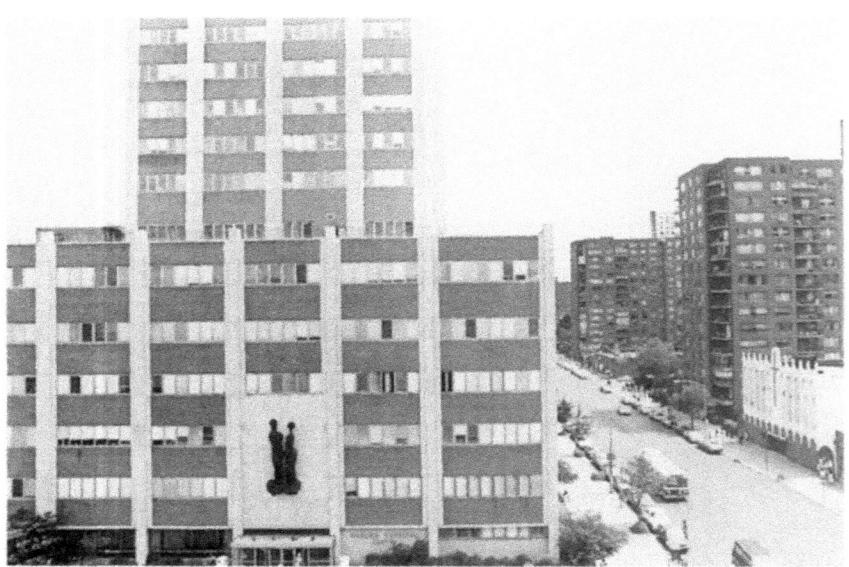

Harlem Hospital Center, New York, New York

Photo Credits

Early Pioneers in Black Psychiatry

Photo	Credit
Walter Adams, M.D.	Courtesy of Howard University College of Medicine
Prince Barker, M.D.	Courtesy of Howard University College of Medicine
George Branch, M.D.	Courtesy of Department of Veterans Affairs, Central Alabama Veterans Health Care System
Herbert Erwin, M.D.	Courtesy of Howard University College of Medicine
Raphael Hernandez, M.D.	Courtesy of Meharry Medical College Archives
Charles Prudhomme, M.D.	Courtesy of American Psychiatric Association Library and Archives
Toussaint Tilden, M.D.	Courtesy of Department of Veterans Affairs, Central Alabama Veterans Health Care System
Ernest Y. Williams, M.D.	Courtesy of Joan Williams-Thomas

Volume Contributors

Photo	Credit
Victor R. Adebimpe, M.D.	Courtesy of Dr. Adebimpe
F.M. Baker, M.D., M.P.H.	Courtesy of Dr. F.M. Baker
James E. Baker, M.D.	Courtesy of Dr. James E. Baker
Bruce L. Ballard, M.D.	Courtesy of *Psychiatric News*
Irma J. Bland, M.D.	Courtesy of Dr. Bland
Clotilde D. Bowen, M.D., F.A.P.M., (L.)APA	Courtesy of Dr. Bowen
Hugh F. Butts, M.D.	Courtesy of Dr. Butts
Joshua W. Calhoun, M.D.	Courtesy of Dr. Calhoun
June Jackson Christmas, M.D.	Courtesy of Dr. Christmas
James L. Collins Sr., M.D., F.A.P.A.	Courtesy of Dr. Collins
Elizabeth B. Davis, M.D.	Courtesy of Dr. Davis
Henry E. Edwards, M.D.	Courtesy of Dr. Edwards

Photo	Credit
Lloyd C. Elam, M.D.	Courtesy of Dr. Elam
John Hope Franklin, Ph.D.	Courtesy of Dr. Franklin
Ruth L. Fuller, M.D.	Courtesy of Dr. Fuller
Tana A. Grady-Weliky, M.D.	Courtesy of Dr. Grady-Weliky
Billy E. Jones, M.D., M.S.	Courtesy of Dr. Jones
Ledro R. Justice, M.D.	Courtesy of Dr. Justice
Mildred Mitchell-Bateman, M.D.	Courtesy of Dr. Mitchell-Bateman
Donna M. Norris, M.D.	Courtesy of *Psychiatric News*
Jeanne Spurlock, M.D.	Courtesy of Dr. Spurlock
Harry H. Wright, M.D., M.B.A.	Courtesy of Dr. Wright

Hospitals

Photo	Credit
Tuskegee Veterans Administration (VA) Hospital, Tuskegee, Alabama	Courtesy of Department of Veterans Affairs, Central Alabama Veterans Health Care System
Freedmen's Hospital of Howard University College of Medicine, Washington, DC	Courtesy of Moorland-Spingarn Research Center, Howard University Archives
Lakin State Hospital, Lakin, West Virginia	Courtesy of Eugene L. Youngue, Jr., M.D.
George W. Hubbard Hospital of Meharry Medical College, Nashville, Tennessee	Courtesy of Meharry Medical College Archives
Homer G. Phillips Hospital, St. Louis, Missouri	Photo by W.C. Persons Missouri Historical Society, St. Louis
Harlem Hospital Center, New York, New York	Courtesy of North Manhattan Network, New York City Health and Hospitals Corp.

CHAPTER **3**

Community Psychiatry and Work in the Public Sector, 1962–1980

JUNE JACKSON CHRISTMAS, M.D.

Looking at community psychiatry and public-sector work in the 1960s and 1970s gives me the opportunity to review my own professional journey. As a psychoanalyst, I realized after nearly a decade of practice that over the years, I might help only a few score persons at most gain an understanding of the complexities of the inner self and thus translate insight into constructive action. I had already broadened my armamentarium beyond the cultural orientation of my psychoanalytic training to include added skills in dynamic psychotherapy and group therapy. As I heard from patients about their lives outside my office and became more aware of the forces contributing to change, I began to work with couples and families. With my mostly middle-class black patients, their dreams, wishes, and actions, grist for the analytic mill, were expressed within the social context. On the other hand, this was not seen with the white patients, who made up the larger proportion of my early years of practice.

When Dr. Elizabeth B. Davis asked me in 1962 to teach group therapy to residents and other staff at the new Department of Psychiatry she was establishing at Harlem Hospital, I was excited at the prospect of this work as a complement to private practice. The department was ripe for innovation and service. As a supervisor, I found it a challenge to help psychiatrists and social workers move from initial doubt about this new technique to become skilled group leaders and open and aware participants in the group process. In the adolescent therapy groups it was a revelation to see the strengths of some of the participants' mothers as they maneuvered their way through the welfare system, or worked two jobs, or stretched their limited budgets. From our successful use of one mother as a volunteer liaison to the school system, the idea occurred to me to use local residents as mental health paraprofessionals. This became a key component in our community psychiatry program for rehabilitating chronically mentally ill black persons in Harlem.

The 1960s: A Time of Social Change

The centuries-old struggle by black Americans for freedom and racial equality gained new energy with the 1954 Supreme Court ruling *Brown v. Board of Education of Topeka, Kansas*. The decision set aside the doctrine of "separate but equal" that had held sway and had enshrined racial inequity in law as well as fact since the Reconstruction. It led to the Civil Rights Movement, the struggle to fulfill the promise of democracy and rid the nation of legally sanctioned racism, segregation, and discrimination. In addition to social activism, the decade was characterized by governmental leadership to redress economic inequities, tentative efforts to provide health and mental health services along a public health model, and citizen participation in decision making. With the press of the Civil Rights Movement and the War on Poverty, human services began to relate to the changing social context. In moving from the traditional focus on treatment of disease alone, health services gingerly began to consider social and environmental factors as forces for the promotion or disruption of health.

Change in psychiatric care was already taking place on several fronts, a continuation of earlier reforms. Across the land, state hospitals increased in size while patients languished on back wards, losing the skills they once had. Often abandoned by families, they deteriorated in an atmosphere of dehumanization and chronicity. The development of psychoactive drugs was a major force for change in individual patients who became free of the gross symptoms of psychosis even though they did not readily regain social skills.

Beginning in the 1950s, a revival of concern about these pitiful conditions had culminated in federal initiatives. The report of the Joint Commission on Mental Health and Illness, "Action on Mental Health," led to the development of a plan for a system of local mental health centers where a range of services would be provided within a neighborhood or catchment area. In the 1960s hundreds of community mental health centers (CMHCs) were set up across the nation with generous federal funding. As so often happens, one of the original major goals was not met—that of linking the new centers with their respective state hospital systems. Generally, the two systems continued separately; often the CMHC was the old wine of the hospital's Department of Psychiatry in a new bottle. Few CMHCs provided the aftercare and rehabilitation that the National Institute of Mental Health initially designated as optional. New demands were made upon our clinics as patients, who were unready to enter community life, were discharged from state hospitals in large numbers. Even though deinstitutionalized, they were in, but not of, the Harlem community. In a different kind of isolation, they lived their lives in single rooms, except when they spent hours sitting in welfare centers or hospital outpatient clinics. Aftercare consisted only of monthly medication at a crowded state hospital clinic; rehabilitation was unheard of.

The Development of the Harlem Rehabilitation Center

Lest these deinstitutionalized individuals inundate the community mental health center planned by the Harlem Hospital Department of Psychiatry, itself in its infancy, I was challenged by the director to design a program to serve chronic patients. She encouraged me to learn about chronic mental illness and add what I discovered to my knowledge of group therapy. Like most New York psychiatrists in private practice then, I found working with persons with chronic psychoses less interesting than working with those with neuroses.

Traveling to other cities, I found few rehabilitation programs. None served black patients in the urban slums. Psychiatrists in these programs worked mainly as dispensers of medications to schizophrenic patients. Even in the successful programs, there was minimal integration of psychiatric knowledge into rehabilitation (Hoffman 1990).

This did not mean that traditional psychiatric therapies were recommended instead. On the contrary, the assumption was that psychotherapy would be ineffective with poor black patients, whether psychotic or neurotic, because "they are not verbal." Even the young black psychiatrists, the core of the new department, expressed doubt about the usefulness of any therapeutic intervention with persons with chronic mental illness. Furthermore, community psychiatry services under the leadership of black psychiatrists were not encouraged. A federal official, justifying governmental reluctance to support such programs, told us that they did not know of any black psychiatrists who had conducted, or could conduct, clinical research. He added that funding any program in Harlem would be "pouring money down a bottomless well."

On one end of the philosophical spectrum, some proffered a social explanation holding the external environment to be the major cause of mental illness. They believed that mental disorders occurred as a result of the detrimental effects of poverty, racism, and discrimination. They maintained that these negative social and environmental factors would first have to be altered—if not eliminated—before one could expect psychiatric services to be effective. Others, aware of the lack of community health services and of community practitioners, urged that the physical needs of people be taken care of before mental health needs were addressed. These narrow views ignored the fact that people in the Harlems of the country suffered from diseases of the mind as well as of the body and that there can be no line drawn separating the human being into a dichotomy of body and mind. These views tended to isolate people from their social environments. We learned that community caretakers and patients expressed a need for both psychiatric and social services. At the same time that developmental policy allowed relative freedom for newer adaptations in social services, there was limited openness to modifications in traditional psychiatric services. There was an openness on the part of the department director to potential program modifications, with the implicit reservation that they remain innovations.

Demonstration projects, pilot programs, and initiation into the world of proposal writing and fund seeking preceded the founding of Harlem Rehabilitation Center in 1964. Located nine blocks from the hospital, it was the first full-range social-vocational psychiatric rehabilitation program in the borough and one of the few in the city. A major grant received from the National Institute of Mental Health (NIMH) provided the funds to renovate two floors of a former factory into a comprehensive multiservice facility and to conduct its programs. From 1964 to 1972, interrelated research grants of $1.92 million supported our studies of the effectiveness of community-based psychiatric rehabilitation with nonprofessional mental health workers as the primary rehabilitative agents. In addition to those from NIMH, funds were provided by the Vocational Rehabilitation Services, the Rehabilitation Services Administration, the New York State Office of Vocational Rehabilitation, and the New York State Department of Mental Hygiene.

Philosophy of Sociopsychiatric Rehabilitation

Because the factors affecting those who are both socially and economically disadvantaged and physically or mentally disabled are so interwoven and complex, no single-faceted rehabilitative approach was thought appropriate to meet their needs. In addition to a multifocused approach, the situation required a different conceptualization of both problem and solution. We developed *sociopsychiatric rehabilitation,* an approach that addresses itself not only to individual educational and vocational potential but also to the economic, social, physical, and psychological factors that enhance or deter the rehabilitative process.

The underlying assumptions of sociopsychiatric rehabilitation were as follows:

- Men and women are valued for their existence and for their efforts toward self-identity, recovery, and self-actualization.
- Human beings, society, and the natural environment are interrelated and interdependent.
- Sociopsychiatric rehabilitation seeks to foster positive change interventions, to increase psychological strengths and adaptive mechanisms, and to use environmental stress to aid individuals to cope more successfully.
- The degree to which an individual's imposed social position has operated disadvantageously in precluding a chance for constructive change must be taken into account.
- Members of the communities related to human-service systems have given high priority to three points of view: as consumers of services; as providers of services; and as participants in the planning, decision making, and control of services.
- The provision of services is a means to constructive change—individual, institutional, and social.

New Careers and New Mental Health Services

The center considered the particular needs of persons who are in positions of marginality because of poverty, illness, psychiatric diagnosis, and race and the alienation and powerlessness experienced as people recover from illness. It used programmatically the lifestyle, language, culture, and labor of black people as they attempted to attain their individual potential (Christmas 1969a).

Most of the patients had had many years of state hospitalization and numerous admissions to public psychiatric hospitals such as Bellevue. Most were poor; occasionally patients were working class or lower middle class.

Only a few had graduated from high school. Before their illnesses, many had low-paying jobs. Most women had been married; many men had not. Most had few remaining family ties.

Early in the process, we modified our original plans to exclude persons with alcoholism from the experimental group. We learned that alcoholism was a secondary diagnosis in 30% to 40% of persons in the outpatient psychiatric clinic and a primary diagnosis in a smaller but sizable number. This observation led to our modifying the research pool and the program. Services for substance abusers increased as the use of illicit drugs spread. In keeping with a holistic approach, we later included persons with a primary physical disability. Most of the patients had the diagnosis of schizophrenia (Jones and Gray 1986; Williams 1986). Every day about 75 to 80 persons attended the two major programs (social and vocational rehabilitation programs). Smaller numbers attended the transitional program and employed clients groups.

In the spirit of the Civil Rights Movement, we tapped the strength of struggle and survival, the beauty of soul, and the essence of the black experience in the rehabilitative process. Patients were known as members in the first stages (the social rehabilitation program and the transitional program) and as clients in the more advanced stages (the prevocational and vocational programs). While recognizing individuality, we believed that group support was a critical change factor. Group approaches were the program's foundation.

The Range of Program Services

The daily programs of 3 to 6 hours were organized along a rehabilitation continuum—social, transitional, prevocational, and vocational. Each program provided health services (medical, psychiatric, and nutritional); social work, community organization, and community action; family casework, counseling, and aid; educational evaluation; literacy training; and remediation activities therapy. Each of the program activities contained varying degrees of key elements that were therapeutic, social, educational, and actional.

All program members/clients and staff participated in center community meetings. Members/clients assumed responsibilities for program activities, self-help groups, and planning. Decision making was shared following therapeutic community principles. Medication groups, with patients providing feedback on themselves and their peers along with staff observations, provided the psychiatrist with more information than the usual monthly visit and was educational as well. Close links with the hospital fostered continuity of care with the Department of Psychiatry and with other departments. Center patients were the first patients at Harlem Hospital to have their own family physicians. The harsh realities of being poor, black, and mentally ill; the struggles seen on television of sit-ins in the South; the school decentralization; and teachers' strikes across the street—these were not viewed as interferences to be eliminated so that orthodox therapy could take place. Instead, they were events that patients and staff dealt with as tasks for discussion, education, coping skills, and empowerment.

Mental Health Workers: New Careers in Mental Health

The small professional staff (psychiatric, social work, nursing, vocational counseling, and educational) took psychodynamics and group dynamics into account in training and supervision of the corps of mental health workers who were the primary rehabilitative agents.

The key to returning to community life was the employment and training of local community residents for innovative roles (Christmas 1969b). We recruited persons in Harlem who had successfully used survival strategies—an honest day's work, hustling, dealing with "the man," breaking the law or abiding by it, or getting the most out of a demeaning welfare system. The aim was to provide employment with dignity, responsibility, and appropriate compensation along with training and education and to provide the opportunity to develop one's own skills and resources and thus advance in a new career. For employment and training as paraprofessional rehabilitation staff, men and women over 30 were recruited through word of mouth, families of patients, tenants and block associations, churches, lodges, welfare and parole office staff, and other formal and informal networks.

In the 1960s, federal funding, although short-lived, was available for paraprofessional training and employment. The principles of new careers included the employment of persons in entry-level positions, acceptance of life experience as a requirement for employment, and the performance of dignified and competent labor with compensation commensurate with duties. Opportunities for upward and lateral mobility and continuing education were also emphasized, as well as meaningful participation in the provision and modification of human services.

Those selected as trainees, through group interviews, showed interest in working with people, empathy, commitment, and general competence. They had the potential to learn to work effectively with groups and individuals and to think analytically. They revealed an openness for constructive self-criticism and personal growth. Experience in, knowledge of, and identification with the lifestyle of the Harlem community was essential. Other general qualifications included: a fifth-grade reading and writing level, formal education limited to high school, the absence of the kind of mental illness that would interfere with functioning, the absence of current substance abuse, the absence of a history of previous employment in mental health, and current unemployment or underemployment.

The trainees had a variety of backgrounds and life experiences. They were homemakers, domestic and factory workers, street-corner men, ex-offenders, welfare recipients, parents, or struggling members of the working class. They represented a cross-section of those who had managed to survive with some manifest degree of strength. It was hoped that this strength and these life experiences would be tapped and used in a process of self-development and service to others. The professional and paraprofessional staff worked in service, research, and training. The professional staff were initially trainers and supervisors. Over two-thirds of the staff were paraprofessionals whose responsibilities varied depending on their programs. Some paraprofessionals were generalists. Others were specialists in health or case services, activities therapies, psychiatric and vocational rehabilitation, education, community organization, or research. A four-step career ladder was projected whereby mental health workers (the eventual title) would advance through trainee, worker, senior worker, and supervisory levels, with advancement recognized by increased responsibility and authority, appropriate work titles, and financial compensation.

Orientation was a full-time learning experience of 6 weeks' duration, using experiential and interfactional approaches. Five weeks were spent in presentations and interfactional discussions, participant observation, sensitivity training, staff meetings, informal peer group discussions, field trips, daily logs, presentations, readings, and evaluation. The 6th week was spent in rotation through center programs.

The in-service training and education program, of 5 to 6 hours weekly, was an integral part of the work situation. It was planned to be carried out over 18 months. It was organized in a way similar to that of the orientation except that the balance of each day was spent in the work situation, under supervision. The six major areas of content were "Core Knowledge of Human Development and Human Services," "Self-Development and Skills Development as a Human Service Worker," "The Black Family: Social Forces, Social Issues and the Human Condition," "The Acquisition and Application of

Knowledge—Techniques of Sociopsychiatric Rehabilitation," "The Use of Supervision and Consultation," and "Supportive Services."

As other programs began to use paraprofessionals, it became clear that there were many explicit and implicit reasons for using local residents for mental health work. We categorized them according to the potential for their activities to contribute to systemic change. These categories are:

- *serving as* a source of low-paid personnel performing menial or low-status tasks
- *playing an aide role,* assisting professionals in performing complex tasks or those simple parts of complex tasks that do not require constant supervision, individual judgment, or initiative
- *providing a communication or cultural bridge* between patients and professionals, helping patients feel more welcome by "adding a little color" to the setting
- *reforming existing systems of service* by the use of new persons in new roles, in limited areas, with limited authority
- *redesigning systems of service,* with a qualitative change in which the helper, the product of a social problem, serves also to help resolve that problem
- *instituting radical change* in a basic restructuring in institutions toward service networks, integration, and collaboration among social systems with staff in new roles, with new responsibilities

Problems and Progress

In its first decade Harlem Rehabilitation Center successfully helped patients become less impaired by their disabilities by returning men and women to constructive lives in the community and by serving in coalitions for social action to improve their living conditions. As a catalyst, it broadened the realm of mental health concern beyond treatment. Its multiservice orientation enriched the practice of medicine and the lives of mentally disabled adults and their families in Harlem.

Evaluation indicated its effectiveness. In contrast to the comparison group of patients receiving standard outpatient services, patients who participated in the center programs showed greater improvement in psychiatric status, measured by structured psychiatric interviews. They also had a greater sense of self-esteem and more social contacts in the community; were more cooperative with medication; had fewer and shorter psychiatric hospitalizations; and were more likely to be involved in work, sheltered work, or school. Lack of housing and jobs for the mentally disabled remained problems, however. These problems were accentuated by the poor quality of absentee-owned housing stock in Harlem, the continuing depressed economic situation, and the persistence of discrimination against people with mental disorders and against black people.

Besides aiding the rehabilitation of hundreds of men and women over the years, the center also helped several scores of men and women to attain economic self-sufficiency as staff in human services and other fields. Some fell by the wayside, victims of the social ills that beset the community. Many more made it in a variety of ways. Some paraprofessional staff used their training and employment to climb up the newly established career ladder in the center, to transfer to other divisions and acquaint them with the new skills of paraprofessionals, and to advance through formal education into the helping professions. A few became professionals, including one mental health worker who finished high school under the program's auspices and eventually obtained a doctorate in social work; she later directed a division at a neighborhood CMHC. Although they are the most dramatic, her achievements should not necessarily be valued by society more highly than are those accomplishments of other paraprofessionals who were able to maintain a meaningful job, finish school, send their children to college, and become contributing community members. Our mental health worker of the 1960s was the forerunner of the case manager for severely and persistently mentally ill persons of the 1980s (Christmas et al. 1970).

The 1970s: Work in the Public Sector in Times of Budget Constraints

The 1970s were a time of contrasts. Militancy and anti-Vietnam and student protests were followed by disillusionment with governmental dishonesty, apathy, and noninvolvement. African American political progress that had begun in the 1960s was not matched by economic progress. Some maintained that we no longer needed programs in which the government was catalyst, initiator, and funder. Withdrawal from social issues, claims that goals of the community mental health movement had been too high, and decreased interest in minority issues predominated (Christmas 1981).

Still, the opportunity I was offered in 1972 to move from program direction to citywide mental health administration was enticing. Perhaps as commissioner of the largest locally administered mental hygiene system in the nation I might be able to apply principles of service to a wider scene, replicate our sociopsychiatric rehabilitation program with other underserved groups, and take part in setting mental health policy.

Planning a Unified Mental Hygiene Service System for New York City

In January 1973, shortly after I became Commissioner of the New York City Department of Mental Health, Mental Retardation and Alcoholism Services, we issued a policy paper that set three goals (Christmas 1973):

1. To develop a single, integrated service system unifying public (state and local) and private (not-for-profit) services, whether preventive, therapeutic, or rehabilitative.
2. To provide care in the least restrictive setting for a defined geographical population, with priority given to populations at risk and with the goal of making quality, effective services accessible, available, and responsive to locally identified needs. Within limits of available resources, the goal was also to ensure that services would be sufficient to meet needs.
3. To include residents of these defined areas and staff members of the institutions and agencies serving these areas in the planning and decision making concerning programs and policies.

The movement toward a locally planned, integrated single system of care—endorsed and affirmed by federal, state, and local governments—had been thwarted by governmental policies that supported fragmentation; by reimbursement policies that encouraged hospitalization; by financing regulations that tended to perpetuate the existing structure and process; and by institutional inertia, often characterized by fear and resistance to change. Most important, the retention of 90% of state funds in a state institutional system while thousands of patients were discharged to local communities and the dual role of the state as funding agency and arbiter on one hand and service provider on the other made progress toward an integrated care system extremely uncertain and rehabilitation services problematic.

The transition from an institutional system to a community-based one was officially proclaimed by New York State but had not been encouraged legislatively, fiscally, or administratively. On the contrary, major obstacles had been imposed. Discharged patients, primarily, were the unfortunate victims. Without sustained treatment and services, monitoring of their medication, and assistance with their domestic and personal tasks, many were unable to cope with unfamiliar chores and unaccustomed responsibilities. They became seriously ill again and had to be hospitalized. Neighborhoods that received substantial numbers of discharged patients were severely affected. Adverse reactions of many communities reflected a long-standing stigma against mental illness. A formidable effort to overcome deep-seated hostilities and fears was necessary.

Yet the local departments of mental health, organized into the statewide Conference of Local Mental Hygiene Directors, continued to press for changes in the system. In 1976, with widespread support and bipartisan efforts, a landmark series of 15 bills represented a vital first step in moving toward comprehensive reform. These bills (state legislation with local support) established a seminal role for the local governmental unit in the process of reforming and integrating services to the disabled, affirming explicitly that the local government is the basic first-stage planning unit for all providers of service, including state facilities and the cornerstone of the anticipated new comprehensive system of care (Christmas 1979). However, the authority for budget allocation of state facility resources still rested with the state. Our department played an active role in these efforts to develop state and local mental health policy. As landmark judicial decisions directed institutions to reduce their size, upgrade the quality of care, and provide minimum standards, civil-liberties issues reinforced the policy of deinstitutionalization. Much-needed community residences and services for the retarded resulted.

It was not so with the mentally ill. An early-action task force on rehabilitation that I established, comprised of providers, governmental agencies, and consumer advocates, produced specific cost-effective recommendations on rehabilitation services for the chronically mentally ill. But, though acknowledging need, city and state budget officials each held the other responsible for funding. Patients remained caught in the middle, with limited aftercare, until Governor Hugh Carey's decision to run for reelection led to a policy of "getting the homeless off the streets." Ultimately state and federal community support system funds came; they were too little and too narrowly defined, but they did lead to resources for rehabilitation and for housing.

However, before the New York City fiscal crisis erupted, the department was able to develop other needed services. We established creative programs in psychiatric rehabilitation, mental retardation, geriatric mental health, alcoholism services (including a program for adolescents), and acute inpatient services in underserved neighborhoods as well as services for children in foster care and the legal system or at risk for severe mental illness. We increased dramatically the number and resources of agencies under the administrative leadership of people of color. We established locally controlled agencies and culturally-specific services in Chinese, Hispanic, and African American communities. With varying degrees of success we pressed for interagency coordination and joint funding. The federation of agencies and consumers that we established played a role in planning and project review that was recognized in the revised state and local law. It also advocated, joined in coalitions, and served as a vocal supporter and critic.

From 1972 to 1975, as commissioner I was project director for an NIMH-funded study of the effectiveness of using the new category of mental health worker throughout the New York City mental health system. This study and earlier research at Harlem Rehabilitation Center formed the basis for new city policies on mental health careers and services. Our efforts resulted in institutionalizing a career ladder for paraprofessional mental health workers in both the civil service and the not-for profit sectors. As project director of 13 community mental health centers and over 90 new programs, I had the ultimate responsibility for designing and implementing the evaluation of these new services as well as of the entire system of over 400 public and not-for-profit hospitals and community-based agencies. It was a challenge to educate agencies, policy makers, and families on mental health and on issues of equity.

Public Policy and Mental Health Issues

Including people of color in policy and decision making does not come easily, even in a department where the leader is also a person of color. Thus, it was necessary for me to meet with management and issue policy statements to reinforce our agency's responsibility for instituting effective equal-employment plans and procedures. At one cabinet meeting, I had to urge a reluctant Mayor Koch to express in a public forum his own commitment to equal-opportunity employment. The difference between equal employment and affirmative action is one of attitude, commitment, and action. My own efforts were to move equal-opportunity employment to a level more consonant with affirmative action. Within the department, we had to show employees how to access both formal and informal complaint procedures. Our inclusion of both minority and nonminority men and women in our functions and communications also sent a message to the rest of the world.

We assisted minority individuals and minority and majority agencies by circulating résumés of minority personnel and lists of agencies and programs. We identified national and local minority organizations in health and human services, organizations with minorities in leadership positions, and organizations concerned with the advancement of minorities. These clearinghouse activities, although carried out on a small scale, often provided search committees or program administrators with information they might not have received otherwise. These activities also served minorities in their need to establish networks to foster affirmative action within their own groups and among these groups, crossing lines that separate ethnic minorities of color and pit them against one another.

The second means by which affirmative action was accomplished was through the development of programs that were culturally and ethnically relevant and that therefore met the needs of particular minority groups. This is especially important when one considers the significance of minority status and the badge of color in a racist society. An ethnic minority individual of color runs a greater risk of being poor and uneducated and of encountering barriers to entering the job market. An ethnic minority family of color is at a higher risk of physical and mental illness, and its access to quality health care is limited.

Yet at the same time, recognition had to be given to the fact that ethnic minorities of color have their own cultural values that should be incorporated as programs are developed to meet their needs. Too often, however, these minorities' coping skills and strengths are ignored as program planners and therapists emphasize the deficit model and identify minority characteristics in terms of their failure to live up to dominant white standards, which are deemed desirable. Both cultural relevance and individual, family, and group coping mechanisms are important. Programs should be developed that are not *in*, but *of*, a particular minority community: community in the sense of neighborhoods where people reside; community in the sense of shared values, relevant to the particular cultural group; and community in the sense of all the residents.

I described six features that should characterize mental hygiene services for ethnic minorities of color: cultural relevance; a holistic orientation; an organizational structure that supports coordination; priority attention to certain target groups (children and youth, the elderly, the formerly and currently institutionalized); the creative use of social and community support systems; and minority involvement in decision making, accountability, and quality assurance (Christmas 1979). As we established alcoholism and mental health programs that used groups and other talking therapies in Spanish family-counseling services or that related to the religious beliefs of black

Americans or to their social clubs, and as we established agencies where newcomers from Puerto Rico were welcomed by people from their hometowns, these programs modified traditional treatment approaches in culturally syntonic ways. Drawing on folk healing—the *curanderos* of Hispanic communities, the medicine men and women of Native American Indian peoples, and the African threads that still persist in black culture—may increase use of services, complement other programs, and make use of information concerning where people customarily turn for help before they seek mental health advice. There was a need for bilingualism in the neighborhoods where newly arrived Chinese lived and in the Haitian communities as well as in other areas, so that people might speak in the language in which they felt more at ease. This is of particular significance in counseling for emotional problems, where communication is vital. Beyond this we encouraged the development of programs that were appropriate to the mores and lifestyles of the particular cultural group, with staff whose sensitivity and knowledge removed what is often a barrier to access to service.

To develop culture-specific models of service delivery meant integrating the positive and constructive values of traditional helpers into less-conventional treatment modalities. It also meant developing an approach that built on social institutions, natural leaders, and community support systems within neighborhoods. To do this, our program developers moved away from what had been an earlier emphasis on traditional psychotherapeutic services, designed for middle-class and working-class whites, to develop a broader array of services to reflect the diversity of New York City. Initially, in the early 1970s, the department urged traditional programs in changing neighborhoods to train their staffs to work with community groups, assisting them in initiating satellite programs that after a period of support would develop autonomous community-based and community-related organizations reflecting changing ethnic needs and under minority control. In black and Hispanic communities, this resulted in the development of freestanding mental health agencies with professionals and paraprofessionals blending their skills with those of the more traditional parent agency. In mental retardation and in mental health, this led to programs that were sometimes linked to poverty programs or community groups (e.g., churches). In other instances, the sponsors were groups with a history of community activism for which this was an initial venture into providing mental health services.

We encouraged the policy that staff of all programs should reflect the range of populations to be served. We were able to follow this policy when it came to recruiting nurses and social workers from the same cultural group as clients. Considering the shortage of psychiatrists in the black community or in the Native American community, however, had we waited until we had the match of ethnicity and patients, programs might not have been started.

Enriching the programs that served minority communities was in itself an affirmative action; assuring that all programs become attuned to the needs of those they serve had the potential to add cultural awareness. But more was required. In the days when money was more available, the department held training programs enabling staff to increase their knowledge and awareness of and sensitivity toward cultural and racial factors. Due to the fiscal crisis, such training was among the programs eliminated in favor of direct services. We continued to encourage programs, particularly the federally funded CMHCs, to use their own funds; some did. Our leadership in conceiving and designing these programs provided an added dimension.

In spite of the budget crisis, we continued to work toward these objectives through our regulatory function. Specifically, to help programs meet community needs and also work toward affirmative action goals, the department required that cultural and ethnic needs be addressed in the annual and long-range plans that we prepared as part of the state service plans. For example, we pointed out to the State Office of Alcoholism Services that with the new interest in alcohol abuse among women, considerable pages in the plans were devoted to women as a group but very little was said about programs specifically addressing the needs of the Hispanic, black, and Native American communities, where alcoholism remained a serious health problem for men, women, and youth.

The Impact of the Fiscal Crisis

By the early 1970s, New York City was experiencing severe financial problems (Christmas 1976). The tax base was eroding as manufacturing and other businesses left the city. Unemployment rates had increased, particularly among young people and minorities. The recession forced more people onto the welfare rolls and placed a heavier burden on the existing human services system. In the eyes of the rest of the country, New York City had caused the crisis by doing too much for its people. What was visible was its extensive public hospital system, its large public education bureaucracy, and its seemingly easy access to public assistance. Less well known was the long-imposed but unusual requirements that the city contribute a portion of Medicaid costs, share in mental-hygiene funding, and fulfill other mandated expenditures.

At the same time that demand for services increased and inflation raised the costs of government, municipal resources were shrinking. A long-predicted crisis was seen as inevitable if these forces continued and outside resources were not made available. Eventually, in late 1975, as New York City teetered on the brink of default, federal and state officials, along with banking and other financial powers, acted reluctantly but decisively. To avoid default, they applied first aid, gave advice, and required cutbacks in city-funded services and programs. Two financial entities were established to monitor and control financial expenditures. As such, the Municipal Assistance Corporation and the Emergency Financial Control Board oversaw the fate of New York City for several years.

As the fiscal crisis intensified, we attempted to protect the innovative minority programs by ensuring that cuts they received were less than those of the larger, more established programs. We never implemented across-the-board cuts or elimination of whole categories of staff. We were critical when hospitals or other large agencies suggested that all their paraprofessional workers be eliminated as a cost-cutting method, one that we maintained would have been detrimental to staff and patients.

Efforts to retain new careerist paraprofessionals within programs had to be supplemented by the department's providing to its contract agencies technical assistance on administration, fiscal affairs, program improvements to remedy the defects that program audits revealed, and recruitment of minority staff. However, because of our own cuts in staffing, we were not able to provide the kind of technical assistance in management that should have been given to the small programs; at times, we found ourselves coming in to ward off a potential crisis rather than being able to stay ahead of the game. This was an extreme problem, because there were some who would rather have seen minority programs go down the drain and, gloating, say "I told you so."

Several large minority community mental health centers with strong clinical staff in executive roles found that they lacked comparable administrative skills. Other programs with dedicated and grass-roots community boards found that without the kind of technical assistance and board member training we tried to provide before the fiscal crisis, board members tended to become involved in day-to-day operations, with negative effects. Other programs, planned before an exodus from a deteriorating community was foreseen, had to develop new ways of reaching out to a diminishing population in the catchment area. The poorest residents, unable to move out of the inner city, had life problems that demanded new types of psychosocial services.

Progress and Problems

In 1976 we looked to a more responsive White House with hope initially but ultimately with disappointment. During this period, in addition to our efforts to increase state aid and to integrate the state psychiatric institutions into a local system of care, we participated in a limited way in efforts to affect national policy. I was asked to head President-elect Carter's transition team developing policy options for the Department of Health, Education and Welfare, the predecessor of the Department of Health and Human Services. Volunteers from across the nation joined our staff; there was enthusiasm that attention would be paid to meeting needs in a more equitable way. Policy analyses prepared by our team looked at plans and impact in what we considered realistic but achievable terms. Disillusionment began when the new leadership showed itself to be willing to go only a short distance into new territories, such as health insurance.

As in the other organizations in which I represented the department, I observed that few black persons were at the table, let alone in the corridors of power. I was often the only person of color who headed an agency and who was thus free to advocate for our needs. The viewpoints of people in black communities and the concerns of the mentally disabled and the poor were rarely raised in the deliberations of the policy makers in charge. When I was approached to head the National Institute of Drug Abuse, I decided that I could better serve minorities and other vulnerable groups by continuing as commissioner; I did, under three mayors, until 1980.

One of President Carter's early acts had been to establish the President's Commission on Mental Health under the leadership of Rosalyn Carter. I was asked to head the work group on community support systems. Here, too, hundreds of volunteers turned their energies to the task of improving mental health systems. After nearly 2 years of diverse participation, the commission recommended reimbursement reform and service integration and gave priority to the chronically mentally ill, children, minorities, and community support. In a ceremony at the White House, President Carter received our reports with thanks but without funds to implement the Mental Health Systems Act. The promise was not fulfilled.

Nevertheless, certain occasions reminded us that the spirit of activism did not die with the 1960s. As budget cuts began to reflect the city's worsening fiscal crisis and the department was threatened by a cut of several million dollars in the city tax levy, a coalition of providers and consumers, led by the mental retardation agencies, mobilized hundreds of people to meet with elected city officials and helped have funds restored. The lack of a constituency had always rendered mental health programs easy prey for budgetary slashes. We sought to expand public knowledge of mental health and enlarge the constituency for the mentally disabled through the media, legislative forums, and community meetings. We learned from consumer members of the federation and parents of the mentally retarded as they taught us how to increase consumer involvement. Recovering alcoholics showed us how to integrate self-help approaches in treatment. We worked with a group of former hospital patients; our pace was too slow for them, and our companions were too deviant for some of our colleagues. But we supported their efforts to empower themselves in the spirit of citizen participation. The problems, though complex, did not seem insurmountable as the 1970s ended.

References

Christmas JJ: Sociopsychiatric rehabilitation in an urban ghetto: conflicts, issues and directions. Am J Orthopsychiatry 39:651–661, 1969a

Christmas JJ: Group methods in training and practice: Nonprofessional mental health personnel in a deprived community, in Psychotherapeutic Agents: New Roles for Nonprofessionals, Parents & Teachers. Edited by Guerney BG. New York, Holt, Rinehart and Winston, 1969b.

Christmas JJ: Issues and directions: The task of providing mental health services in New York City. Presented at Gracie Square Hospital, New York, New York, January 17, 1973

Christmas JJ: The fiscal crisis and its impact on mental health services in the Bronx. Presented at the Bronx Rotary Club, Bronx, New York, November 16, 1976

Christmas JJ: Progress and problems along the road to a single service system. Psychiatry Ann 9:82–83, 1979

Christmas JJ: The challenge of change. Am J Public Health 71:235–241, 1981

Christmas JJ, Wallace H, Edwards J: New careers and new mental health services: fantasy or future? Am J Psychiatry 12:464–476, 1970

Hoffman JS: Integrating biologic and psychologic treatment: the need for a unitary model, in Psychiatric Clinics of North America. Edited by Marcus E. Philadelphia, PA, WB Saunders, 1990, pp 369–372

Jones BE, Gray BA: Problems in diagnosing schizophrenia and affective disorders among blacks. Hosp Community Psychiatry 37:61–65, 1986

Williams DH: The epidemiology of mental illness in Afro-Americans. Hosp Community Psychiatry 37:42–49, 1986

CHAPTER 4

Development of the Department of Psychiatry at Meharry Medical College

LLOYD C. ELAM, M.D.

This chapter focuses on the persons and events that contributed to the establishment of a department of psychiatry at a historically black medical school in the United States. Particular attention is directed to the recruitment of faculty, development of a clinical service and outreach to the community, development of a curriculum of particular relevance to black students, and the community's ambivalence about psychiatry.

Meharry Medical College was established in 1876 with a mission to educate black doctors who would go back into the communities to serve. The institution was begun as a medical department of Walden University, which was associated with the Methodist Church. Because of an interpretation that charitable foundation funds could not go to schools that were associated with organized religion, and because the hierarchy of Walden University wanted to remain associated with the church, the medical school became independent of Walden. This set the groundwork for Meharry Medical College as an independent body.

Prior to the development of the Department of Psychiatry there was no psychiatric service at Meharry. All students rotated at Homer G. Phillips Hospital (St. Louis, Missouri) for their clinical work. Meharry faculty assumed the responsibility for the didactic work in psychiatry. When Robert S. Anderson, M.D., assumed the directorship of the Department of Medicine, he advised the dean of the School of Medicine, Daniel Rolfe, M.D., and the president of the college, Harold D. West, Ph.D., of the growing importance of psychiatry and the need for a department of psychiatry.

67

In a school with a special mission, the dynamics are affected by the tremendous changes in community expectations and changing opportunities as well as by the changing science and methodologies taking place in the field. When the special mission involves serving the black community, the ambivalence of that community as well as of the wider community becomes a part of the equation because resources and expectations come from the different extremes. In the case of psychiatry, the ambivalence is related to issues of race and poverty and the question about the proper place of psychiatry. The question is answered differently in different times in different communities.

The ambivalence is shared by physicians, patients, financial institutions, and the general public. Physicians are skeptical about whether many of the disorders dealt with in psychiatry are real illnesses in the first place and, if they are, whether they respond to psychiatric interventions other than medication. Despite this skepticism, psychiatry owes its existence to the physicians who recognize that among the most frequent maladies affecting mankind are phobias, depressions, anxiety disorders, and other disorders that indicate some function of the brain is overperforming, underperforming, or being applied incorrectly. Because psychiatry depends on the other physicians for its existence, attacking this skepticism has not laid to rest the question of the real place of psychiatry in the scheme of things.

Skepticism by physicians plays into the hands of the patients, who, because of denial, guilt, or lack of understanding, would rather see their discomfort as resulting from external stress, supernatural forces, or some physical malfunction that does not involve the brain or the mind. This may explain why patients wait for excessively long periods before seeing a psychiatrist, even in the face of severe suffering. Community beliefs, as well as the unavailability of psychiatric treatment, have been known to foster denial. Knowledge about the outcome of nontreatment (e.g., suicide, missed days from school or work, hazards of self-medication with alcohol) has not eradicated the skepticism.

Ambivalence and denial have always been manifested in a lack of adequate funding and the assumption that other professionals and nonprofessionals could do the job of caring for the psychiatric patient. Shifting the categorization of the psychiatric disorder is another factor that warrants consideration. The shift may lead to a recategorization into the "corrections" arena, or simply the roles of the unsuccessful. Another approach to dealing with behavior due to psychiatric disorder is to define or categorize it as criminal behavior or simply the behavior of the unmotivated and unsuccessful, thus shifting the responsibility away from the medical field altogether.

Despite all the alternative methods used to serve the mentally and emotionally ill, because of increases in numbers of mental hospitals it was perceived that there was an increase in the number of the mentally ill during the half century before 1960.

The Recruited Chair

The usual recruitment techniques were unsuccessful, but Dean Rolfe would not abandon the idea of securing a chairman and psychiatrists to establish a department of psychiatry at Meharry. During a meeting in Chicago, he discussed the matter with Dr. C. Knight Aldrich, then the chairman of the Department of Psychiatry at the University of Chicago. They proposed a plan to select and groom a black psychiatric resident. At the time, I was a psychiatry resident at the University of Chicago; Dean Rolfe and Dr. Aldrich approached me about the position. Although my interest was provoked immediately, several questions surfaced. Why would I want to leave Chicago with all of its needs, challenges, and opportunities to go to an area where the challenges were certainly evident but where few recognized the need? Furthermore, there were uncertainties about the availability of a support system and about the expected patient population. Would it be expected that psychiatric services focus primarily on black patients with psychotic disorders?

I could see some advantages as well. For example, the smaller city could be more suitable for family life and raising children. The opportunity to design a program to meet the needs of the black population was appealing. At Meharry, as perhaps at no other place, I could help bring the new developments in psychiatry to medical students who had identified a primary care specialty as a career choice. I would also have the chance to share this information with other health care students and health care providers (e.g., nurses, dentists, physicians) who were members of the faculty or had maintained a close relationship with Meharry.

The offer of the position was a once-in-a-lifetime opportunity. The interest displayed by the head of the department of medicine, the dean, and the president played no small part in assuring me that a support system could be developed at Meharry.

During the last months of training, I took advantage of every opportunity to learn about administration. One such opportunity was an elective offered by Dr. Aldrich, who was assisting in setting up a new service at the recently established Illinois State Psychiatric Institute. I made frequent trips to Nashville to participate in planning the new psychiatry department, which initially would consist of an inpatient service and offices.

During this period it was not yet popular for a black family with origins in the South to return there, and I felt some trepidation about moving into a southern community that was more segregated and perhaps more discriminatory against blacks than Chicago had been. But this was the time of Civil Rights activity, and Nashville provided an opportunity to be involved in history-making events.

Challenges That Faced the New Department Chairperson

It was perhaps a culmination of the aforementioned factors that provoked my excitement about going to Meharry to establish a department. I, along with my very supportive wife, a registered nurse, saw the problems as opportunities and took the inconveniences in stride.

In September 1961 in Nashville, a member of a church in the black community called the police to report that a black man was arguing with the men of the church and disturbing the peace. The police came and fatally wounded the man. Because there was no mental health center or mental health service in the community for the police to look to as a source of help, no one was able to report whether he had been psychotic, or intoxicated, or homeless.

Meharry Medical College decided to establish a department of psychiatry in 1961, and in September of that year I arrived to assume my new position. The president of the college had obtained a $25,000 grant as seed money for the development of the department. Plans called for adding a wing to the hospital to house the new department. My excitement about the potential of the department overshadowed the problems. Timing was the first obstacle. The construction of the new wing had not proceeded on schedule and was far from completion at the time that psychiatric services were to be instituted. This problem was viewed by me as a minor inconvenience. Of more concern was the fact that the board had decided, prior to my arrival, to discontinue the nursing school. This was fairly significant; the opportunity to teach psychiatry in the nursing school had been a major attraction for me in considering the position.

Atmosphere

Despite the aforementioned problems, which could be looked upon as merely speed bumps along the road, there was considerable excitement about the new department. Students and faculty were warm and supportive; I had no question as to whether I had made the right decision. As an example of the willingness to be helpful, the student government association, which had only two offices, was willing to turn over one of them to me until some renovation could take place. Almost all of the persons who had been psychiatry lecturers agreed to continue and to be involved in planning curriculum changes. Hospital staff readily agreed to reassign the holding area (which had been used to retain patients while arrangements were being made to transfer them to the state hospital) to the new department.

Focus on Decision Making

What kind of department should be developed in the black medical school? Should it be like the departments in all other medical schools? Should it be fashioned to meet the needs of the patients and the students? Or should research be the primary focus in the planning? With some discussion from faculty members and the absence of research support, I determined that the main focus of the department would be to teach students, who would later be general practitioners and specialists; to recognize and treat or refer psychiatric patients; and to participate in the training of nurses and other personnel in the care of psychiatric patients. The education of psychiatrists would not be the primary concern of the department, although I recognized that some training of psychiatrists would take place. The provision of inpatient and outpatient services would also be central in the planning.

Equally important was changing the image of the institution, which had in the past been dependent on part-time faculty from other institutions. In keeping with the activities of the Civil Rights movement, self-reliance would mean developing independence as a major mission, not only in obtaining grants for training and research but also for contributing to the development of self-reliant services. The paradox is that the more independent an entity, the more necessary it is for that entity to interact with others. To achieve its goals, Meharry was required to interact with other educational, service, financial, and political entities both inside and outside the college; it was an opportunity to be a part of the change and, in some cases, to lead it. A big order for a small department, perhaps, but being small was not one of the goals.

The Curriculum

In the medical school the teaching program had consisted of lectures in personality development and psychopathology, followed by a month's clinical experience during the third or fourth year. Around the 1960s and before, the curriculum consisted primarily of preparing students for a psychodynamic understanding of psychiatry and lectures in personality theory, the doctor-patient relationship, sociological aspects of mental and emotional illnesses, and diagnosis of these illnesses. Clinical experience was primarily related to the diagnosis and care of inpatients. These activities were embellished by participation in medical and surgical grand rounds and occasional clinical pathological conferences in which the psychiatrist could make meaningful contributions. The drugs used in the treatment of the mentally ill at that time were primarily Thorazine, Compazine, Sparine, and a few other antipsychotic medications. Librium and meprobamate were used for anxiety, and the one drug available for depression was imipramine. The curriculum included teaching students about the action of these drugs and their use for mentally ill and emotionally disturbed patients. A great deal of the emphasis was placed on psychotherapy and the management of the psychiatric patient.

With the new department, it would be necessary to alter the curriculum in order to equip students with a knowledge base for dealing with populations whose cultural backgrounds were not white middle-class. Whereas textbooks and general psychiatry were based on studies of the majority population, Meharry served blacks from all socioeconomic levels as well as poor whites. What were the characteristics of those populations that would affect the mental and physical health of members of each group? The idea that people in different cultures were biologically different certainly was not an adequate explanation. The change in the curriculum required more emphasis on sociology, anthropology, psychology, and the role of religion while giving adequate coverage of nutrition, sexuality, and lifestyle. Psychology and aspects of the doctor-patient relationship remained the strongest emphasis. Teaching the biological basis of psychiatry had always been the responsibility of the basic science departments of the medical school. This did not change; however, the support of the Department of Psychiatry provided additional lectures to strengthen the core.

Just as the preclinical curriculum was changed, the clinical experience would also be modified to address the challenges a physician could expect. Rather than being based entirely in an inpatient setting, students were exposed to outpatient services and consultation to medical and surgical outpatients. The curriculum allowed the student with special interests, including research, to spend some time in other learning environments.

The curriculum committee was very cooperative in providing time for lectures in the preclinical years and for demonstration or supervised therapy during the clinical years. Special experiences had to be scheduled during the summer months. With the new curriculum in place, it was possible for a student to have some exposure to behavioral sciences or psychiatry during each quarter of the year. Although psychiatry was used as a part of the forward thrust in medicine and faculty members from other departments felt a part of this thrust, they were reluctant to give up curriculum time from their own departments. Therefore, the curriculum committee felt some reluctance to giving the time requested for the newly proposed curriculum for psychiatry. The students were pleased with the changes in the curriculum; however, many of them perceived psychiatry as the "icing on the cake" rather than as one of the core disciplines that they needed to master in order to become doctors.

Faculty

During the early years of Meharry, much of the teaching in all the disciplines was done by Vanderbilt faculty. Until 1961, psychiatry was a division of the Department of Internal Medicine. Except for Dr. Raphael Hernandez, who served on the faculty in the 1930s and 1940s until he was drafted into military service, and Dr. William Silcott, who served in the 1940s and 1950s, lectures in psychiatry were usually delivered by part-time faculty, who also served as consultants. Much credit is owed to Dr. Hernandez (sketches of his professional career are outlined in Chapter 1 of this book), who taught neurology, anatomy, and neuroanatomy as well as psychiatry. The psychiatric services were coordinated by a social worker, Betty Sarpe.

The establishment of a department meant reliance on full-time faculty for teaching. The circumstances at Meharry attracted and retained faculty who were willing to face challenges and accept an opportunity to serve others in the absence of great material rewards. Early in the life of the department, I was fortunate to recruit the following individuals on a full-time basis:

Henry Tomes, Ph.D., a graduate in psychology at Pennsylvania State University, was one of the prime movers in the development of the Community Mental Health Center.
Evelyn Kennedy, R.N., a major teacher in the new curriculum, recruited the staff for the inpatient service and led the establishment of the first day hospital program in the state.

Ralph Hines, Ph.D., a sociologist at Howard University, joined the faculty as medical sociologist and vice chairperson of the department.

Charles Proctor, Ph.D., a behavioral pharmacologist who had been studying biological aspects of schizophrenia, joined the faculty to teach biological aspects of psychiatry.

Raphael Hernandez, M.D., rejoined Meharry as a member of the faculty of the Department of Psychiatry.

Gunstav Batizy, M.D., joined the faculty as clinical instructor in 1963.

Audrey Wall, M.S.W., filled the position vacated by Betty Sarpe's resignation and geographical move.

Addressing the Ambivalence About Psychiatry

Treatment of patients in their natural settings was the strategy used to combat the fear and prejudice that some members of the community had demonstrated about mental illness. With this in mind, psychiatrists made house calls, and treatment in the day hospital was emphasized. Instead of using entry-level attendants, students from the local theological seminary and psychology students from a nearby university were recruited for training and service on the inpatient unit. Thus, residents from the nearby community became familiar with psychiatric patients as members of humankind and in turn became strong supporters of the psychiatry program.

Research

During the formative years of the department, teaching and service responsibilities did not allow the small faculty time for conducting research. Nevertheless, the faculty encouraged and supported students' interest in research endeavors. Early in the functioning of the department, the research of two students was particularly outstanding. Marion Bowers was engaged in a research project on monoamine and anxiety disorders. While still a student, he presented a paper on his work at a meeting of the Southern Association of Psychiatry. He went on to pursue an academic career but transferred his interest to otolaryngology. Gloria Johnson Powell, who became nationally known for her research on psychiatric aspects of school segregation and desegregation, began her work when a student at Meharry.

Summary

The Department of Psychiatry at Meharry began its journey in 1961. As a young recruit, I joined the faculty and, with the assistance of faculty I recruited, built a department that was successful in the school and in the community. I went on to become dean and president of the college, and the department continued its development under successive chairpersons.

Additional Readings

Bulletin of Meharry Medical College. Vol 55, No 4, 1959
Meharry Medical Bulletin. 1960–1964
Summerville J: Educating Black Doctors. The University of Alabama Press, 1983

CHAPTER 5

Participant Observer: The Experiences of a Black Transcultural Psychiatrist

VICTOR R. ADEBIMPE, M.D.

Introduction

A doctor coming from Africa to train as a psychiatrist in the United States would seem to have many adjustments to make personally and professionally because of the wide differences in social, cultural, and political world views between his origins and his destination. In reality, Western medicine and its traditions have been the basis of medical school education in most parts of Africa. The adaptations necessary for competent functioning as a professional are not so great. However, a black doctor who arrived as I did in 1972 would have come to America shortly after the founding of the Black Psychiatrists of America, which was formed to address the effects of prejudice on the mental health care of black Americans (Pierce 1974).

My thanks are due to several individuals who helped with my work and provided much-needed support and teaching at crucial times. I am particularly grateful to Alice D. Kitchen, M.D.; James L. Hedlund, Ph.D.; Richard C. Evenson, Ph.D.; Carolyn Kruse, R.N.; Sobhana Mehta, M.D.; Dinesh Mehta, M.D.; Helen Klein, D.S.W.; Tyler Person, M.A.; Horacio J. Fabrega Jr., M.D.; Samuel M. Turner, Ph.D.; David J. Kupfer, M.D.; Susan Edwards, M.S.W.; Fred Fowler, Ph.D.; Linda Falorio; Roy Lahet; Richard J. Rach; Beverly Smith, R.N.; William H. Wilson, Ph.D.; Frank E. Sessoms, M.D.; the late Charles J. Burks, M.D.; Lois Dabney-Smith, Ph.D.; James H. Carter, M.D.; Jeanne Spurlock, M.D.; Michael Reardon, MBA; Delores Parron, Ph.D.; Tony Strickland, Ph.D., and Lisa Green, M.D.

The officials of the National Institute of Mental Health (Ochberg and Brown 1973) conceded that:

1. National admission rates to both inpatient and outpatient psychiatric facilities are higher for nonwhites than for whites;
2. Nonwhites show minimal use of private psychiatric facilities;
3. Puerto Ricans in New York State constitute 9.1% of first admissions to state schools for the retarded, whereas their proportion to the whites of the state population is only 4%;
4. The 1960 census indicated that 48% of institutionalized nonwhites lived in hospitals and homes for the physically and mentally handicapped while 80% of institutionalized whites lived in such facilities. In contrast, 49% of the nonwhites were in correctional institutions compared with only 16% of whites. These data suggest vast inequities in the handling of behavioral problems of persons of different social and racial backgrounds (p. 571).

To a black immigrant psychiatric resident, such facts were both disquieting and challenging. Disquieting because they shattered my hopes, based upon my experiences as a medical student in Africa and Great Britain, that the United States was the best place in the world to study mental disorder in black patients. It now seemed merely the least of several evils. Particularly disturbing was the following assertion by a team of well-informed experts at the National Institute of Mental Health:

> Racist practices undoubtedly are key factors, perhaps the most important ones in producing mental disorder in blacks and other underprivileged groups, in determining the place where members of these groups receive diagnosis and treatment for these disorders, and in determining the quality of such clinical services. . . . accounting wholly for or at least in part for the epidemiological differences reported (Kramer et al. 1973, pp. 355–356).

The challenging aspect had to do with the fact that in the late 1960s and early 1970s controversy raged over the reliability of data used to support the notion of a higher rate of mental disorder among blacks, an idea that dates back more than 100 years. Thomas and Sillen (1972), Pasamanick (1963), and Fischer (1969) faulted these data because they were drawn from public mental hospitals that admitted more indigent patients. The researchers pointed out that these patterns were given more credence than they deserved probably because of the long-standing need to depict blacks as mentally inferior and thereby justify slavery. Related questions had also been raised about the mental functioning and the distribution of mental disorder among blacks in Africa and in Great Britain: Does the stress of racism cause any difference in the epidemiology of various psychiatric disorders? Is the low incidence of depression found in American blacks similar to that reported for Africans? Were there reliable statistics of schizophrenia and depression corrected for age, sex, and social economic factors, all of which were well known to significantly modify such statistics? Are psychological tests more objective for blacks than clinical diagnoses? Are lower IQs in American blacks a reflection or validation of the assessment by British psychiatrists of lower intellectual ability in Africans? Are there personality differences that support or refute similar assessments of impaired frontal lobe functioning in Africans?

Are mental differences found between blacks and whites compounded by the ways blacks are treated by mental health systems . . . in other words, are these systems, in effect if not in intent, discriminatory?

At first, I thought people simply did not want to talk about these questions, wondering why I was so inquisitive about such a sensitive matter. I quickly learned, however, that even those who knew that I was asking these questions to prepare myself for my future work in Africa did not seem to have any reliable answers. Worse still, neither did the books written on the subject. They too were full of questions that were unanswerable because of the rudimentary stage of the techniques of psychiatric diagnosis and psychiatric epidemiology.

I wondered how it was possible on one hand to document the fact that there were no reliable figures for the prevalence of mental disorder in the community, while at the same time asserting that such data as were available were influenced by racist practices. My impression was that it was quite likely that not every institution was culpable in all the alleged areas and that there might be some way of separating pervasively discriminatory systems from those that were innocent or merely partially deficient in some areas.

Resolution of Scientific Controversy, 1974–1984

All things considered, the most important questions seemed to be: 1) Is there evidence for a pattern for unintended inequalities? 2) Is there any evidence for malicious motivation associated with such patterns? 3) Is it possible to identify rectifiable inequalities and thus separate them from intractable ones?

These questions were simple to ask but not easy to answer. Some of them were difficult to bring up in discussion, much less to analyze. At first

I was dismayed by the lack of information on these issues in textbooks and by the ignorance of my teachers beyond what they knew as lay individuals. It was obvious that very few persons could help me in the task of analyzing even the concrete scientific aspects of these questions, not to mention the tangled political dimensions of some of them.

But I reminded myself of the Yoruba proverb:

Owo ara eni l'aa fii
Tun nkan ara eni se.
(Translation: The best help
Is self-help.)

For some time, self-help meant interminable debates between the naturally biased black, the knowledge-hungry resident, and the agnostic epidemiologist. To really understand the questions, specific areas of clinical psychiatry, psychology, sociology, anthropology, epidemiology, and statistics had to be mastered.

Later, I decided to research these questions rather than endlessly debate them. I was particularly fortunate to have at my disposal the computerized records of patients in public hospitals and clinics in the state of Missouri, which were routinely stored at my residency training institute in St. Louis. It was possible to use such a database to compare symptoms and signs of psychiatric disorders in groups of black and white patients matched for age, sex, years of education, and income: an important step if one is not to be misled by spurious differences in the two ethnic groups.

Researching Diagnosis of Depression in Blacks

In the late 1960s depression was widely reported to be less frequent in African societies than in the West (Leighton et al. 1963; Prince 1968). In the United States clinicians believed that this condition was rare among blacks. I was particularly struck by the similarity of psychosomatic symptoms of depression between American and African blacks and the report by Carter (1974) that it was this presentation of depression rather than its frequency that was different. It also seemed understandable that if, as was hypothesized, some kinds of abnormal behavior (e.g., alcoholism, drug abuse, sociopathy) were "depressive equivalents" among blacks, the diagnosis of affective disorder would be made less frequently among them, a proportion of cases receiving these other diagnosis labels instead.

My colleagues and I were able to match 49 pairs of depressed black and white patients for age, sex, and socioeconomic status. Surprisingly, differences among patients were quite modest and somatic symptoms were similar in both groups (Adebimpe et al. 1982b). This confirmed the findings of other investigators in which, after correction for the aforementioned demographic variables, no black-white differences existed in patients diagnosed with depression or mania (Helzer 1975; Tonks et al. 1970). There seemed to be no reason for the symptoms to mislead clinicians into diagnosing another disorder when evaluating depressed black patients and thereby generating statistics showing a lower frequency of this condition among them.

Researching Overdiagnosis of Schizophrenia in Blacks

In 1974, it was not easy to make that simple statement. Black psychiatrists asserted that black patients were overdiagnosed in some categories and underdiagnosed in others, most likely because white psychiatrists misinterpreted symptoms and other behaviors in black patients. Considering the rudimentary state of psychiatric diagnosis for any ethnic group at that time, the evidence for this assertion was scanty, but I could not help being impressed by two particular investigations.

A research study done at nine New York state mental hospitals required research psychiatrists to use structured mental status interviews to diagnose patients whereas hospital psychiatrists used their routine interview methods. In spite of lack of differences in the psychopathology shown by black and white patients, the hospital clinicians diagnosed schizophrenia more often and affective disorder less frequently among the blacks. The structured interview used by research diagnosticians found no ethnicity-based differences (Simon et al. 1973). This pattern was also shown in an even more extensive study involving 159 black and 555 white depressed patients. Blacks were diagnosed as schizophrenic reaction, schizoaffective type, whereas whites were more likely to be diagnosed with psychotic depression (Raskin et al. 1975). Some confirmation of these patterns was found in another study in which researchers rediagnosed with computer algorithms a group of patients to whom a clinical impression had been assigned by clinicians (Welner et al. 1973).

I decided to study the possible explanations for these patterns, which none of these researchers had offered. I had the opportunity to make firsthand observations relevant to this problem during my work as a research psychiatrist on a study of the clinical and social characteristics of black and white schizophrenic patients in urban and rural settings in Missouri. This was part of a transcultural research study comparing the factors associated with the relapse and readmission of schizophrenic patients in Turkey and the United States (Adebimpe et al. 1981; Adebimpe et al. 1982a). The data were collected using structured interviews administered by nurses, social workers, and psychiatrists on admission, discharge, readmission, and follow-up. Two hundred seventy-three patients consecutively admitted to seven hospital and mental health centers over a 3-year period were rated by the research team. The frequency of auditory and visual hallucinations was higher among black patients, but delusional symptoms appeared with the same frequency. Many other symptoms were different between the two groups. For example, black patients were more angry, impulsive, dysphoric, and asocial. In reviewing the research literature we found that hallucinations and delusions had been reported more frequently among blacks and that this may include patients who were not necessarily suffering from a psychosis. For example, one report showed that among the normal adults of a southern black community, young females reported frightening hallucinations along with phobias and emotional distress, whereas elderly males reported tranquil, placid, and often hypnagogic hallucinations. I inferred therefore that a baseline of nonschizophrenic hallucinations among blacks underlay the higher frequency of this symptom among black schizophrenics and that such hallucinations may mislead the unwary clinician into diagnosing schizophrenia in otherwise normal individuals, or those whose psychosis derived from affective disorders, alcoholism, organic brain syndromes, and hysterical states. This inference was supported many years later among black patients with dementia in New York and black schizophrenic patients in Great Britain. Hallucinations were found at a higher frequency in both samples and could mislead unwary clinicians to diagnose schizophrenia among the patients suffering from dementia. A higher frequency of the same symptoms among black schizophrenics, compared with their white counterparts, seemed to reflect a baseline of hallucinations separate from those indicating schizophrenic psychopathology. In both situations the use of structured diagnostic instruments guided the clinicians to arrive at the correct diagnosis (Cohen and Carlin 1993; McGovern et al. 1994).

Researching MMPI Diagnosis of Black Patients

In further attempts to account for possibly spurious higher rates of schizophrenia I also reviewed the possible effects of inaccurate psychological tests in influencing the diagnostic thinking of clinicians. This was only a few years after the publication of Jensen's (1969) article regarding the relatively low IQ scores of blacks, and various critiques of his questions were still being hotly debated by those who insisted that few psychological tests were standardized on the typical inner-city black person and that the validity of most tests for blacks was dubious.

I wondered if any of the tests then used involved any such bias and reviewed the Minnesota Multiphasic Personality Inventory (MMPI), which had scales for both depression and schizophrenia and caught my attention because of the findings of Simon et al. (1973) and Raskin et al. (1975), described earlier. The review of the literature showed that the majority of a sample of normal rural blacks were labeled schizophrenic by this instrument and that this pattern was found among psychiatric patients. One study recorded that 60% of black psychotic patients in contrast with 44% of whites were inaccurately diagnosed by the MMPI. I inferred, therefore, that false or exaggerated diagnoses of schizophrenia by MMPI testing may influence clinicians to confirm their erroneous diagnosis with the presumed greater scientific validity of the MMPI, and that this may partly account for the higher rates of schizophrenia reported for blacks. I cautioned that clinical psychologists should make interpretations that take into consideration the possibility of falsely elevated scales, and also that psychiatrists should be aware that false positive diagnoses are a distinct possibility and that test reports that are at variance with other clinical information should be given special scrutiny (Adebimpe et al. 1979). These comments remain valid more than 15 years later, since other tests show arbitrary black-white differences (Hamberger and Hastings 1992), and the MMPI has had to be redesigned to take into account the problems associated with the ethnic diversity of test takers (Butcher et al. 1990).

Researching the Basis for Scientific Controversies

The aforementioned investigations did not completely answer the question of the distribution of mental disorders among both ethnic groups. In studying this problem I was impressed with the many pitfalls awaiting anyone who wished to do an in-depth analysis of it, and therefore I was able to appreciate and understand the alternative positions for each controversy. The various phases of race relations had shaped the choices of research topics. The climates of opinion clearly influenced the interpretation of data. Objectivity suffered from the constant topicality. Some topics, especially intelligence, had traditionally been discussed in terms of superiority and inferiority, with ethnocentric interpretations of black-white differences and their implications for public policy. Many variables studied were shown to be determined more by age, gender, and socioeconomic status than by ethnicity, but the necessary statistical corrections for these factors were not always made, causing investigators to find dubious ethnic differences and to draw unwarranted inferences. There was often confusion about the anthropological use of the word "race" when it was used interchangeably with "ethnicity."

Given these constraints, it was difficult to properly assess the validity of most of the data purporting to show black-white differences in the presentation and distribution of mental disorders. Particularly puzzling to me was the number of admittedly methodologically imperfect studies that seemed to show no ethnic differences. Considering the extra psychosocial stresses that blacks experience, I thought this would mean that even though the more vulnerable individuals might succumb to such stresses (as in suicide), the vast majority of blacks seemed to possess coping skills that prevent chronic negative emotions from developing into psychiatric syndromes. I pointed out that the epidemiological facts needed to be verified and that the relevant coping skills should be studied for use in counseling and perhaps in suicide interventions (Adebimpe 1984). My own prediction and bias was that there was no obvious basis for expecting an ethnicity-related difference in the distribution of most mental disorders, but that I would be more reassured by retrospective studies of data collected from multiple sites for investigations with no obvious racial implications so as to eliminate parochial and observer biases (Adebimpe 1984). Such studies did not appear in the literature for almost 10 years. But when they did, they were a clear confirmation of that prediction (Adebimpe 1993; Kessler et al. 1994; Robins and Regier 1991).

Meanwhile, I was able to make a few additional relevant observations from my experience of patients coming into psychotherapy. At first, I did not know what to make of the literature on blacks in psychotherapy. Some investigators found the race of the therapist to be critical for successful outcomes, whereas others reported that therapeutic skills were more important. For some time it was fashionable to recommend specific training of white therapists to improve their competence in bringing cultural awareness to psychotherapy. Poverty and social class, in addition to ethnicity, were obstacles in access to psychotherapy and also tended to militate against blacks being able to obtain maximum benefit from counseling. I had the opportunity to confirm all these observations in two clinical settings. From 1987 to 1992, as medical director of Charles R. Drew Community Mental Health and Mental Retardation Center in Philadelphia, where 85% of patients were black, I was able to observe that retention of black patients in psychotherapy was definitely higher than what was reported in other settings. It was my impression that in this predominantly lower-class population, therapy tended to focus on how to cope with unemployment, violence-ridden neighborhoods, housing problems, sexuality in the age of AIDS, and juvenile delinquency rather than on traditional white middle-class mental health problems. Client and therapist satisfaction with usual therapy concerns seemed somewhat elusive and seemed to hinge upon success in accomplishing concrete goals in the aforementioned areas.

Recognizing that difficulties with patient-therapist empathy and rapport place severe limitations on the levels of self-disclosure a black patient can attain when talking to a white therapist, I devote a large portion of my psychotherapy practice to black patients to provide an opportunity for more candid communication. In this setting I have had many black patients referred to me who indeed had issues that would have been difficult to bring up and explore in a regular employee assistance program office. A recent client, a 32-year-old black male, was referred to me with the diagnosis of paranoid schizophrenia because he complained of discriminatory practices on his job as a machinist at a local factory. Eight prior years of near-perfect attendance and positive job performance did not protect him from this diagnosis. He was full of rage not only at the events that led to his being referred to his company doctor but also about the psychiatric diagnosis. Both combined to produce persistent homicidal thoughts and plans directed toward specific authority figures at the factory. He had expressed fears of "going off and hurting someone" but had said nothing about wanting to kill somebody until he came to my office. Since he showed no evidence of schizophrenia, I stopped his neuroleptic medications. There was no emergence of schizophrenic symptoms for 18 months. At the end of that period the patient's company insisted on an independent evaluation in order to settle his case. A detailed and otherwise competent assessment produced another diagnosis of paranoid schizophrenia despite the absence of hallucinations and delusions or paranoid behavior outside the work setting. This case illustrated the misinterpretation of symptoms and was a situation in which self-disclosure of potentially explosive impulses would be less likely with a white clinician (Adebimpe 1981, 1982).

This example is not at all uncommon and is a variation of the theme of misdiagnosis partly because the patient was overly hesitant in giving sensitive details of the history to a white therapist and partly because a diagnostician did not fully appreciate the difference between a victim's fear in a threatening situation and paranoia when there are few or no stimuli. It is therefore not surprising that many blacks turn to traditional caregivers and to indigenous churches before considering formal psychotherapy or psychiatric consultation.

The diversion of a significant proportion of black patients to such alternative sources of care may contribute to the lower rates of affective disorders reported for them in national statistics. It also indicates that some responsibility for suboptimal utilization of available clinical resources lies with the black community.

My success in satisfying my scientific curiosity about the issues discussed here, and in resolving some of the controversies (at least for myself), was helpful in decreasing some of the feelings that I had at the beginning of my training. Others were not so easily satisfied. I was irritated that these controversies were not being seriously addressed by professional organizations to which I belonged, and I missed having the stimulus that would have been thus provided by studies confirming or refuting my findings. I felt some embarrassment that I was researching issues that many psychiatrists refrained from talking about. This feeling was heightened by my African concept of good manners, which is summarized in a Yoruba saying:

A kii ti oju onika mefa kaa.
(Translation: If your host has six toes,
don't count them aloud.
Meaning: Don't go on and on about
your host's congenital anomalies.)

Then there was my own fear that I might uncover facts about which I would be uncomfortable, such as confirming or being unable to refute speculations by earlier investigators that amount to a psychological trident for individuals in the black diaspora—which was and still is a real threat to the self-image of anybody who is persistently given the feedback that he or she is deficient in intelligence, personality, and mental functioning. Realizing that my natural bias could always stand in the way of my efforts to arrive at a scientifically valid opinion about many of my research questions, I insisted on methodological rigor and conceptual economy, especially because opportunities for epidemiologic studies were usually few and far between.

These feelings and considerations caused me to hesitate in proceeding with my investigations, but they were overcome by even stronger feelings of compassion for several individuals who would suffer from inadvertent inequalities if these issues were not researched and clarified. I felt that it was more a technical problem with political overtones rather than the other way around. I hoped to discover a method for rational evaluation of alleged disparities in mental health delivery and a scientific approach to eliminating them. In the 1970s, both were badly needed, not only in the United States but also in Great Britain and South Africa (Don 1981; Jewkes 1984; Littlewood 1993). The cooperation that I received from several key persons in carrying out my research was quite remarkable and unusual, considering the nature of my topic, the constantly changing climates of interracial relations, the understandable defensiveness of many organizations regarding such research, and the premature timing of some of it with regard to the sophistication of psychiatric diagnosis and epidemiology. It is to the credit of the scientific climate in this country that any of my work was performed, much less published.

Progress Notes, 1972-1997

Race, Racism, and Mental Disorder

A 1993 letter to the editor of the *American Journal of Psychiatry* shows that some of the technical issues of diagnosis and treatment of blacks remain outside the awareness of many who should be knowledgeable about them, if only for clinical competence. The author concluded that "there is no valid clinical reason for the patient's race to hold the prominence it now does in case presentations," even though he conceded that sensitivity to social issues, including issues about race, would be helpful in making clinical decisions (Porter 1993). This letter thereby ignored recent reviews of the literature that indicated that thousands of publications show a tendency for making racial comparisons for diseases associated with promiscuity, underachievement, antisocial behavior, sexually acquired diseases, suboptimal intellectual performance, drug abuse, violence, and sexual assault (Osborne and Feit 1992). It also ignored the significance of the Epidemiologic Catchment Area study (Robins and Regier 1991), which after adjustment for various demographic variables showed quite unimpressive ethnic differences in the community prevalence of mental disorders, laying the responsibility for differences observed in the hospitals and clinics at the doorstep of mental health care delivery systems and providing a surprisingly precise answer to the long-standing universal and controversial questions of the relationships between race, racism, and mental disorder.

In 1994 I documented an array of clinical situations in which inequalities in the experiences of blacks and whites were undeniable. Some of these were expected and probably acceptable whereas others were not. Deliberately perpetuated inequalities are, in my experience, far less common than those based on technicalities that can be measured, modified, and monitored (Adebimpe 1994b).

If there are little or no racial differences in the epidemiology of mental disorders in the community but hospital and clinic statistics show large differences in many areas, "a method for rational evaluation of alleged disparities—and a scientific approach to eliminating them," without much argument or debate were, at last, feasible. It was finally possible to suggest new clinical standards and deflect emphasis from the relatively sterile explanation of "racism." Examples of inequalities were in the areas of health-seeking behavior, voluntary and involuntary commitment, inclusion in research samples, psychiatric diagnosis, psychological tests, psychotherapy, and responses to certain medications. Clinicians can rectify most of these by paying greater attention to clinical policies and procedures regardless of their personal attitudes toward black patients.

Any institution in which such inequalities cannot be demonstrated would have a good chance of successfully countering charges of racial discrimination. Persistent patterns of inequalities, on the other hand, are easily discoverable by a retrospective review of clinical records. Patterns of care that are inconsistent with public policy as expressed in the nondiscrimination statements prominently displayed in the lobbies of most hospitals and clinics can then be monitored by such bodies as the Joint Commission for the Accreditation of Hospitals, Medicare, and third-party payers, all of whom have an interest in not paying equally for unequal care. Collecting data necessary for monitoring patterns of care to other American minorities by this method is now a major research challenge (Adebimpe 1994a).

Attention to such areas of clinical management may render some of the debates that have been reported in Great Britain (Littlewood 1993) a matter of comparing black-white differences in retrospective data corrected for age, sex, and socioeconomic status. Patterns of differences that emerge after such adjustment can then be compared with data of community prevalence, which to the best of my knowledge has yet to be collected in Great Britain on a national scale comparable to that of the Epidemiologic Catchment Area study. If, when such surveys are conducted, no racial differences are found, this would call for closer scrutiny of the pathways that make possible some of the wide black-white disparities reported in case registers. Substantial differences in the community, on the other hand, could provide fertile clues for the etiology of schizophrenia and affective disorders.

Sufficient data for a fair analysis of reports of inequalities in apartheid South Africa were not available in the published literature (Jewkes 1984), but improvements are being promised in the near future (Urquhart 1994).

Race and Intelligence

Some progress, though not much, has been made in the interpretation of IQ tests in the past 20 years. In the early 1970s, Jensen's controversial article (Jensen 1969) in which he inferred like others before him that blacks were inferior to whites in abstract problem-solving ability but equal or superior to them in rote learning and memorization was hotly debated. Some authorities argued for caution in drawing this type of conclusion from the available data, maintaining that the concept of race is more demographic than anthropologic. Black psychologists called for a moratorium on testing black children and tried to develop test batteries that they believed were more likely to reflect black culture. In my practice, I routinely added 10 points to a black patient's calculated IQ to see if the result was more congruent with the clinical presentation. Even if this was an error, it was on the side of greater rather than lower expectations for the patient.

Noting that the intellectual, artistic, and technological achievements of the various races demonstrate their broad capacities when performing under optimal conditions, I commented that in the examinations conducted for high school graduating classes by the universities of London and Cambridge for the British Commonwealth, national racial or ethnic differences had not been highlighted. I further stated that

> although IQ testing is useful for discovering which individuals or ethnic groups need various educational subsidies, the effects of racism make the United States a poor and elusive laboratory for studying the relationships between race, ethnicity, and intellectual performance. (Adebimpe 1984)

Herrnstein and Murray (1994) revived this debate in their book *The Bell Curve: Intelligence and Class Structure in American Life*. I no longer had the feeling of loneliness in grappling with a technical problem that had political ramifications. It was gratifying to see a wide variety of commentators stating that even if the facts of racial differences were beyond dispute, public policy is a choice that must be rooted in sound scientific reasoning rather than alarmist reinterpretations of old data (Browne 1994; Herbert 1994; Holt 1994; How Clever Is Charles Murray? 1994; Lieber 1994; Melloan 1994; Morganthau 1994; Staples 1994).

It should be self-evident that regardless of the actual differences in group means of IQ scores, it is in the interest of American society to put in place whatever educational and vocational subsidies are necessary for every individual to achieve the maximum level of functioning and quality of life that is possible for his or her level of mental ability. It is appropriate to recognize, acknowledge, and appreciate efforts made in this direction in the past three decades. Relentless reanalysis of group differences should not detract from the primacy of this goal, and divisive predictions should be seen as a challenge for greater creativity in attaining it. A boosted IQ may or may not be one of the side effects of this task. An excessive valuation of what IQ tests measure could mean a dangerous devaluation of all the things that they do not measure but could contribute to the good life, the good society, and the highest quality of life for all. Suboptimal success in the attainment of this goal after the first efforts should not be a cause for discouragement and might even be expected during a transitional stage on the way toward a clearly articulated social destination. The necessary attitude may be found in a Yoruba proverb:

Irorun eiye
Ni irorun igi.
(Translation: The birds are at peace
when the tree in which they nest is at peace,
the tree is not at peace if the birds are not at peace.
Meaning: Mutual nurturance is an ecological imperative.)

The bell curve becomes a bell curse only if society ignores the fact that mutual nurturance is an ecological imperative.

Race and Violence

Other perceptions of blacks, also rooted in myths from the past, are more difficult to analyze. A good example is the notion that blacks are inherently more violent than whites and that there may be a genetic explanation for such a difference. A major controversy over this issue resulted in the cancellation of an NIMH conference in 1993 and was related to that institute's director being relieved of his position because comments he made about inner-city black males were thought to be insensitive and inappropriate for a high-level public official (Scheck 1993; Williams 1994).

The minimum requirements of a plausible hypothesis for a genetic basis of black-white differences in violence would seem to be 1) a black-white difference in the frequency of unambiguous indicators of violence, after correction for age, gender, socioeconomic status, and handling by the criminal justice system; 2) a higher prevalence of violent behavior in the relatives of convicted felons of either ethnic group; and 3) a black-white difference in the community prevalence of the psychiatric disorders most closely associated with violent behavior (i.e., sociopathy and schizophrenia). Clear demonstration of such phenotypical differences might be a logical theme for further research studies before public funds are committed to the search for a corresponding genotype, especially in that there is no indication that "violence" is genetically encoded in the same way as schizophrenia, bipolar disorder, or other mental disorders.

The debate continues, showing that scientists are sometimes unaware that the opinions they hold as laypersons may have been acquired in ways quite different from those their professional standards dictate.

Diversity in Health Care

The preceding discussion notwithstanding, it is good to be able to say that these issues are receiving attention at the highest levels of government and that the attention given to them in the early 1970s was not merely a transient response to the racial strife of the late 1960s. In March 1994, new guidelines published by the National Institutes of Health urged researchers to set up outreach programs to recruit minority and female patients who might otherwise be underrepresented in clinical trials, so that statisticians can accurately analyze whether treatments affect these subpopulations differently. Researchers were also encouraged to break out data on subpopulations rather than group them in categories so unwieldy as to be almost useless.

Greater attention is now being paid to situations where blacks receive inferior care compared to whites despite equal access to medical care and equal ability to pay for medical services, indicating that social class differences may not explain all the disparities. For example, in a Veterans Affairs Medical Center study involving 33,641 males, blacks received substantially fewer cardiac procedures after acute myocardiac infarctions than whites (Peterson et al. 1994). Paradoxically, they had better short-term and equivalent intermediate survival rates compared to whites. Similarly, the quality of hospital care for insured Medicare patients was found to be influenced both by the patient's race and financial characteristics and by the type of hospital in which the patient received care (Kahn et al. 1994).

Considering the odds, Americans have every reason to be proud of the progress that has been made in narrowing the gaps in the delivery of mental health care to blacks and whites in the past several years (Livingston 1994; Adebimpe 1997) and of the example they have set for other countries.

References

Adebimpe VR: Overview: white norms and psychiatric diagnosis of black patients. Am J Psychiatry 138:279–285, 1981

Adebimpe VR: Psychiatric symptoms in black patients, in Behavior Modification in the Black Population. Edited by Turner SM, Jones RT. New York, Plenum, 1982

Adebimpe VR: Overview: American blacks and psychiatry. Transcultural Psychiatric Research Review 21:81–109, 1984

Adebimpe VR: Race and crack cocaine (letter). JAMA 270:45, 1993

Adebimpe VR: Clinical and research challenges in the diagnosis and treatment of mental disorder in ethnic minorities. Presented at the second annual Conference on Psychopathology, Psychopharmacology, Drug abuse and Culture. Los Angeles, October, 1994a

Adebimpe VR: Race, racism, and epidemiological surveys. Hosp Community Psychiatry 45:27–31, 1994b

Adebimpe VR: Mental illness among African Americans, in Ethicity, Immigration, and Psychopathology. Edited by Al-Issa I, Tousignant M. New York: Plenum, 1997, pp 95–105

Adebimpe VR, Gigandet J, Harris E: MMPI diagnosis of black psychiatric patients. Am J Psychiatry 136:86–87, 1979

Adebimpe VR, Klein HE, Fried J: Hallucinations and delusions in black psychiatric patients. J Nat Med Assoc 73: 517–520, 1981

Adebimpe VR, Chu CC, Klein HE, et al: Racial and geographical differences in the psychopathology of schizophrenia. Am J Psychiatry 139:888–891, 1982a

Adebimpe VR, Hedlund JL, Cho DW, et al: Symptomatology of depression in black and white patients. J Natl Med Assoc 74:185–192, 1982b

Browne MW: What is intelligence and who has it? New York Times Book Review, October 16, 1994, p 3

Butcher JN, Graham JR, Williams CL, et al: Development and Use of the MMPI-II Content Scales. Minneapolis, MN, University of Minnesota Press, 1990

Carter JH: Recognizing psychiatric symptoms in black Americans. Geriatrics 29:95–99, 1974

Cohen CI, Carlin L: Racial differences in clinical and social variables among patients evaluated in a dementia assessment center. J Natl Med Assoc 85:379–385, 1993

Don AM: More on the South African report. Am J Psychiatry 137:866, 1981

Fischer J: Negroes and whites and rates of mental illness: reconsideration of a myth. Psychiatry 32:428–446, 1969

Hamberger LK, Hastings JE: Racial differences in the Millon Clinical Multriaxal Inventory in an outpatient clinical sample. J Pers Assess 58:90–95, 1992

Helzer JE: Bipolar affective disorder in black and white men, a comparison of symptoms and familial illness. Arch Gen Psychiatry 32:1140–1144, 1975

Herbert B: Throwing a curve. The New York Times, October 26, 1994, p A15

Herrnstein RJ, Murray C: The Bell Curve: Intelligence and Class Structure in American Life. New York: The Free Press, 1994

Holt J: Anti-social science? The New York Times, October 19, 1994, p A3

How clever is Charles Murray? The Economist 333:2–30, 1994

Jensen A: How much can we boost I.Q. and scholastic achievement? Harvard Educational Review 39:1–60, 1969

Jewkes R: The case for South Africa's expulsion from international psychiatry. New York, United Nations Centre Against Apartheid, 1984

Kahn KL, Pearson ML, Harrison ER, et al: Poor hospitalized Medicare patients. JAMA 271:1169–1174, 1994

Kessler RC, McGonagle KA, Zhao S, et al: Lifetime and 12-month prevalence of DSM IIIR psychiatric disorders in the United States. Arch Gen Psychiatry 51:8–19, 1994

Kramer M, Rosen BM, Willis CV: Definitions and distribution of mental disorders in a racist society, in Racism and Mental Health. Edited by Willie CV, Kramer BM, Brown BS. Pittsburgh, PA, University of Pittsburgh Press, 1974

Leighton AH, Lambo TA, Murphy JM, et al: Psychiatric Disorder Among the Yoruba: A Report of the Cornell-Afro Mental Health Research Project. Ithaca, NY, Cornell University Press, 1963

Lieber M: An anthropological look at race and intelligence. Chicago Tribune, October 23, 1994, section 4, p 13

Littlewood R: Ideology, camouflage, or contingency? Racism in British psychiatry. Trans Psychiatr Res Rev 30:243–290, 1993

Livingston IL (ed.): Handbook of Black American Health: The Mosaic of Conditions, Issues and Prospects. Westport, CT: Greenwood Press, 1994

McGovern D, Hemmings P, Cope R, et al: Long term follow up of young Afro-Caribbean, and White Britons with a first admission diagnosis of schizophrenia. Soc Psychiat Psychiat Epidemiol 29: 8–19, 1994

Melloan G: The "Bell Curve" sells genetic science short. The Wall Street Journal, October 31, 1994, p A15

Morganthau T: I.Q.: is it destiny? Newsweek, October 24, 1994

Ochberg FM, Brown BS: Key issues in developing a national minority mental health program at NIMH, in Racism and Mental Health. Edited by Willie CU, Kramer BM, Brown BS. Pittsburgh, PA, University of Pittsburgh Press, 1973, pp 555–579

Osborne NG, Feit MD: The use of race in medical research. JAMA 267:275–279, 1992

Pasamanick B: Some misconceptions concerning differences in the racial prevalence of mental disease. Am J Orthopsychiatry 33:72–86, 1963

Peterson ED, Wright SM, Daley J, et al: Racial variation in cardiac procedure use and survival following acute myocardia infarction in the Department of Veterans Affairs. JAMA 271:1175–1180, 1994

Pierce CM: The formation of the black psychiatrists of America, in Racism and Mental Health. Edited by Willie CV, Kramer BM, Brown BS. Pittsburgh, PA, University of Pittsburgh Press, 1973, pp 525–554

Porter JL: The use of race in case presentations. Am J Psychiatry 150:1129, 1993

Prince R: The changing picture of depressive syndromes in Africa. The Canadian Journal of African Studies 1: 177–192, 1968

Raskin A, Crook TH, Herman KD: Psychiatric history and symptom differences in black and white depressed inpatients. J Consult Clin Psychol 43:73–80, 1975

Robins LN, Regier DA (eds): Psychiatric Disorders in America: The Epidemiologic Catchment Area Study. New York, Free Press, 1991

Scheck A: Crossing the line: pickets protest meeting on mental disorders and ethnicity. Clin Psychiatry News, February 1993, pp 1–13

Simon RJ, Fleiss JL, Garlans BJ, et al: Depression and schizophrenia in black and white mental patients. Arch Gen Psychiatry 28:509–512, 1973

Staples B: The scientific war on the poor: the ugly politics of I.Q. New York Times, October 28, 1994, p A18

Thomas A, Sillen S: Racism and Psychiatry. New York, Brunner/Mazel, 1972

Tonks CM, Paykel ES, Klerman GL: Clinical depressions among Negroes. Am J Psychiatry 127:329–335, 1970

Urquhart C: Ending medical apartheid. Am Med News November 7, 1994, p 1

Welner A, Liss JL, Robins E: Psychiatric symptoms in white and black inpatients, II: follow-up study. Compr Psychiatry 14:483–488, 1973

Williams J: Violence, genes, and prejudice. Discover, November 1994, pp 93–102

CHAPTER 6

Black Americans in Military Psychiatry

CLOTILDE DENT BOWEN, M.D., F.A.P.M., (L.)APA, COL.
U.S. ARMY (RET.)
JAMES L. COLLINS SR., M.D., F.A.P.A., COL. U.S. ARMY (RET.)

Since the armed forces began training black American psychiatrists in the 1960s, several have served as career military psychiatrists, and others have made significant contributions to military medicine during periods of active and reserve duty. Throughout the years of racial segregation in our armed forces, black military personnel had to overcome numerous obstacles to achieve significant positions of responsibility. This chapter provides a brief account of the first black physicians to serve in the military and the more recent experiences of black military psychiatrists.

In "Black Defenders of America," Major (Ret.) Robert E. Green (1974), U.S. Army, reported that black American physicians were first used in the U.S. armed forces during the Civil War. Several thousand have served with distinction since that time, and to date three have earned the rank of brigadier general in the regular United States Army Medical Corps: Brigadier General (Ret.) Guthrie Turner, M.D., Brigadier General (Ret.) Vernon Spalding, M.D., and Brigadier General George Brown, M.D. Several others have earned the rank of flag officer in the medical corps of regular, reserve, and National Guard units.

The Civil War

The first known black American commissioned medical officer in the army was Lieutenant Colonel John Van Surly deGrass, M.D. (Collins 1974). He served as an assistant surgeon with the 35th Infantry Regiment U.S. Colored

Troops. At the war's end in 1865, seven other black American physicians were on active duty. They were recruited to help care for the 180,000 black American servicemen who served in that conflict. These physicians were Charles Purvis, Alpheus Tucker, John Rapier, William Ellis, Anderson Abbott, William Powell Jr., and Alexander Augusta.

Major Martin Delaney, M.D., was a Harvard-trained physician but was commissioned as an infantry officer. He was personally recruited by President Lincoln to enlist recently emancipated slaves to join the Union army during the final months of the Civil War (Cornish 1966).

World War I to Vietnam

During World War I, 365 black physicians served on active duty. At the conclusion of World War II, more than 600 were serving around the world, and 143 served during the Korean War. Two hundred served during the Vietnam conflict. The exact number of black American physicians who have served on active, reserve, and National Guard duty to date is unknown because the services no longer keep racial statistical data on physicians. The numerous contributions and achievements of these men and women will never be known until their as yet untold stories are adequately recorded by military historians and in the popular media and press.

Black American Psychiatrists in the Military

In attempting to collect data for this chapter, the authors learned that there are no official records that identify military psychiatrists by race or ethnicity. Making use of the oral tradition of black people and a review of membership directories of the American Psychiatric Association, we were able to identify close to two dozen black American psychiatrists who served in the reserves of one of the branches of the armed forces or as careerists in the military.

The first known black American psychiatrists trained by the army were Leo Oxley, Jay Randall, Henry Edwards, James L. Collins Sr., and Thomas Guyden (all M.D.s and captains).

Other black psychiatrists who are known to have pursued psychiatric training at Walter Reed Army Hospital include the following: Dewitt Alfred, Edward Baldwin, Tonya Cheevers, James Thomas Howard, George Milton Lewis, Jerome Massenburg, William R. Mays, Enid Sheeley, James Almer Smith III, Gaston Stewart, Fern J. Thomas, Benjamin Walker, and Michael Wymes. Those who are known to have been affiliated with the U.S. Navy include Vivian Campbell, Floyd Charles, Claude Coleman, Vince Dillan, William Forte, Lillian Fuller, and Regie Givens.

From our search we determined that fewer black psychiatrists were active members of the air force. George Hudson, Frank Hayes, Leonard Lawrence, and Ledro Justice are included in this group.

What Do Military Psychiatrists Do?

Many of the psychiatric problems seen in service members, their families, and retirees are very much like those found in civilian populations with similar demographic characteristics. Some of the emotional problems associated with war and its aftermath, however, are unique to military psychiatry.

Military psychiatrists are assigned to various service facilities—some near combat zones, others in facilities stateside and abroad. The following sampling of assignments is illustrative:

Dewitt Alfred—medical officer, USAF Regional Hospital, Chanute Air Force Base, Illinois; psychiatric services at Andrews Air Force Base, Maryland, 1967–1968; chairman, Department of Mental Health, Regional Hospital, Sheppard Air Force Base, Texas, 1968–1971

Jocelyn Bonner—staff psychiatrist, psychiatry service, 67th Evacuation Hospital, USA, Wurzburg, Germany, 1988–1991, and chief, 1988–1991

Clotilde Dent Bowen—assistant chief, psychiatry and neurology, chief, psychiatry service, Tripler General Hospital; chief, psychiatry outpatient service, Schofield Barracks, Hawaii, 1967–68; director, Review Branch, special assistant for psychiatry, OCHAMPUS, Denver, CO, 1968–1970, 1976–1977; chief, psychiatry, Tripler Army Medical Center, Honolulu, Hawaii, 1974–1975; commander, Hawley U.S. Army Clinic, post surgeon, psychiatric consultant, U.S. Army Study of Women in the Army, Ft. Benjamin Harrison, Indianapolis, IN, 1977–1978; chief, primary care (including general outpatient clinic, emergency, and 5 outlying health clinics in Utah and Colorado), Fitzsimmons Army Medical Center (FAMC), Denver, CO, 1978–1983; chief, psychiatric consultation service, FAMC, Denver, CO, 1983–1985

James L. Collins—chief, psychiatry, Tripler Army Medical Center, 1986–1988; Commander, U.S. Army Hospital, Vicenza, Italy, 1988–1990; Commander, U.S. Army Hospital, Berlin, Germany, 1990–1992; Commandant, F. Edward Hébert School of Medicine, Uniformed Services University of the Health Sciences, Bethesda, MD, 1992–1996; chief, Department of Psychiatry, Walter Reed Hospital, Washington, DC, 1996

Frank Hayes—chairman, Department of Mental Health, David Grant USAF Medical Center at Travis AFB, 1966–1968; chairman, Department of Mental Health, U.S. Air Force Hospital, Lakenheath, England, 1968–1972; chairman, Department of Psychiatry, Uniformed Services University of the Health Sciences, Bethesda, MD, 1976–1979

Ledro R. Justice—chief, psychiatry service, 11th U.S. Air Force Hospital (PACAF), Thailand, 1974–1975; psychiatrist, Mental Health Clinic, USAF Hospital, Lakenheath, England, 1975–1977; psychiatrist (1977–1979) and chief (1979–1980), Mental Health Clinic, USAF Medical Center, Andrews AFB, Washington, DC; chief, mental health services, USAF Regional Hospital, March AFB, CA, 1980–1982

Leonard E. Lawrence—chief, child guidance clinic, Wilford Hall USAF Medical Center, Lackland AFB, Texas, 1969–1972

James Almer Smith III—chief, inpatient psychiatry, Womack Army Hospital, Fort Bragg, North Carolina, 1980–1981; chief, outpatient psychiatry, Womack Army Hospital, Fort Bragg, North Carolina, 1981–1982; served in Operation Desert Storm/Desert Shield, 1982

Michael Wymes—chief, child psychiatry service, 121st Evacuation Hospital, 1984–1986; assistant chief, inpatient psychiatry service, Letterman Army Medical Center, San Francisco, CA, 1987–1989; chief, consultation liaison service, Letterman Army Medical Center, San Francisco, CA, 1990–1991; chief, child and adolescent psychiatry service, Community Mental Health Service, MEDDAC, Fort Belvoir, Virginia, 1992–1994

The lack of complete confidentiality between the psychiatrist and the service member undergoing treatment frequently causes many service personnel and their families to avoid necessary treatment because they fear that the stigma of psychiatric illness may hamper the service member's career. This is true in the case of certain individuals, such as ambitious, higher-ranking personnel and others who require security clearances; however, for the majority of service members, confidentiality is adequately maintained. Military psychiatrists must maintain the physician-patient relationship and at the same time represent the company they work for—the U.S. government. One of the authors (CDB) recalls the dilemma some military psychiatrists experienced when stationed at Fort Leavenworth Kansas in the early to mid-1970s. At that time, if an officer or a member of his or her family overindulged in alcohol or engaged in spousal or child abuse, or if the teenagers were using marijuana, drinking, breaking curfew, or acting out sexually, the family kept their problems under wraps until the inevitable "family explosion" that almost always resulted in the end of the officer's career. To preserve confidentiality, one army psychiatrist either never saw families of these officers at the mental health clinic or minimized incriminating notes on the chart. Some families sought psychiatric services in the local community. Many of the career army officers attending the command and staff college felt that no family problems were permissible if they were to have successful careers; problems had to be kept within the family and could not be shared with military psychiatrists. Today, the lack of total confidentiality of service members remains a concern to many service personnel and is presently being addressed in civilian courts.

Combat Stress Behaviors

Combat stress behaviors may be adaptive or dysfunctional. The most serious of these behaviors are those involving criminal acts. It has been noted that all combat stress behaviors evolve into posttraumatic stress disorder (PTSD) (Jones 1995). During exposure to prolonged combat, fear of death and mutilation in battle can cause even the bravest soldiers to become dysfunctional. It has been observed, however, that one battle's coward may become the next battle's hero. For many years, military leaders have searched for a process of selecting the soldiers who are the most mentally and physically fit for combat. To date, no reliable selection process has been developed to weed out all soldiers who may develop dysfunctional combat stress behaviors.

In September 1942, more service members were evacuated from the armed forces for psychiatric disorders than were inducted in that month. The drain of potential manpower was obvious, and military leaders decided to reexamine the policy of eliminating service members who showed any sign of anxiety, depression, or mild to moderate emotional symptoms. Military psychiatrists were assigned to field units and put into practice some of the techniques used in previous wars to reduce the mass evacuation of psychiatric casualties.

After these techniques were perfected, as many as 70% of soldiers suffering from symptoms of battle fatigue could return to military duty within

72 hours. The treatment principles were proximity (treat close to the front lines but remove soldiers from direct enemy fire), immediacy (treat right away), expectancy (let soldiers know that they are not patients and are expected to return to duty), and simplicity (provide sleep, hot food, showers, clean clothes, and supportive counseling). The staff continuously reinforced the expectation that soldiers would return to duty. The soldiers often referred to the treatment as "three hots [meals] and a cot [sleep]."

In today's wars, battle fatigue and combat stress reactions are still inevitable when hundreds of thousands of soldiers are required to go to war. Many service personnel will succumb to the stress and horrors of the modern battlefield just as they have done throughout history.

"Three hots and a cot" did not work as well in the Vietnam War, which had shorter, less-intense battles and few static battle lines. This war was a guerrilla war, and the soldiers did not manifest the classical symptoms of battle fatigue. Instead they presented with problems of alcohol and substance abuse, disciplinary infractions, and "self inflicted" medical disorders such as malaria (brought about by failure to take prophylactic medications). As the neuropsychiatric consultant to the Vietnam theater surgeon, Bowen learned that combat stress treatments learned in previous wars could not always be effectively applied in the Vietnam combat zone. Soldiers were often sent on search-and-destroy missions close to 100 miles away from the home base to locate Viet Cong guerrillas. If they developed dysfunctional combat stress symptoms on these missions, no mental health help was nearby.

Bowen also observed that other soldiers were sent in helicopters on commando-type missions of several days' duration to isolated areas of Vietnam. Some combatants brought their dead back to base camp after a firefight. Sometimes they had to load the dead on planes that were headed to the United States. After several days, some soldiers developed dysfunctional combat stress symptoms associated with handling dead bodies. Brief treatment was not always beneficial, and many of them had to be evacuated home.

Some of these soldiers had also "self-medicated" on drugs and alcohol and were emotionally numbed and cognitively impaired. They felt that drugs and good luck were their only hope to get them through their 365-day combat tour unscathed. If they were unlucky, they would go home in body bags or be maimed and return as wounded casualties. Unfortunately, many were evacuated back home to "the world," as they called it, as substance-abuse psychiatric casualties. Bowen noted that by the end of 1971, during their tours of duty in Vietnam, more than 400 soldiers per month required drug detoxification. The problem became so acute that it could no longer be ignored by the brass and families back home, because the soldiers wrote about the widespread drug use in Vietnam and talked about it on their return to the States. Many soldiers began to use amphetamines and other controlled substances to stay "macho" and to control their fear and boredom.

The stateside antiwar sentiment came to Vietnam with the new recruits. Many of them failed to carry out their military duties and ended up in military jails, on drugs and fighting each other. The incidence of dysfunctional combat stress symptoms increased among the soldiers, and for many, jail was a better alternative than dying in combat.

Medical personnel also developed signs and symptoms of PTSD, although they often "positively adapted" to combat stress by taking care of patients. For some, their own repressed combat stress symptoms turned up much later. Both authors admit to their own delayed physical and emotional symptoms following their war experiences. Excerpts from Bowen's war memoirs describe her adaptation to her year in Vietnam:

> As the neuro-psychiatric consultant, I travelled extensively all over Vietnam in helicopters, and was exposed to enemy fire . . . I spent nights in bunkers, alone and afraid, as we were shelled or rocketed by the enemy . . . . Once on a mission, through enemy territory, to visit troops at a firebase, our helicopter was hit by ground fire, but we managed to land safely . . . Although frightened, I had to fly over enemy territory again and again.
> . . . later, I flew over a battle, near the demilitarized zone in the Brigade Commander's helicopter, while Air Force B-52 bombers dropped their bombs from five miles up . . . I rode in jeeps at night, through enemy held territory, to visit a hospital near the Viet Cong controlled, infamous village of My Lai . . . I was forced to land in a busy airfield in a plane with no radio, or contact with the tower, by helping the pilot watch out for other planes taking off and landing. I warned the pilot that an Air Force plane was taking off straight towards us. . . . yes, I was often exposed to death, but not on a daily basis . . . Finally one becomes numb, and the delay in instituting treatment no longer seemed to affect me or many of the other psychiatrists.

As a psychiatric resident at Walter Reed Army Hospital from 1969 to 1972, Collins was on the receiving end of the hundreds of casualties generated by Vietnam. His memoirs reflect experiences similar to those of Bowen.

> Sometimes the medical evacuation plane landed at Andrews Air Force Base full of psychiatric casualties. We were assigned as many as 30 patients each, and the five psychiatry wards were always full. Many of the patients were psychotic and had symptoms of auditory and visual hallucinations. In those days we did not yet know much about substance abuse with amphetamines and other drugs, and many patients were initially diagnosed as having schizophrenia. As they rapidly improved, however, we realized that they were not schizophrenic but were suffering from amphetamine and other organic psychosis. The soldiers told us that they bought the drugs over the counter

from Vietnamese pharmacists under the trade name of "obesitol," a French diet control pill. Most of these patients were discharged from the hospital and returned home, but a few had lingering flashbacks about their traumatic war experiences.

During the last year of formal training the seven senior residents at Walter Reed expressed some concern and anxiety about the possibility of assignment to Vietnam. Collins recalls feeling that

> I was one of the lucky ones, and did not have to be separated from my wife and two young children, but I never got over my survivor's guilt about not going to Vietnam, even after my unlucky resident-mate returned safely when the war ended.
> ... I will never forget the double amputees or the head injured youth who never woke up, or the burn victims whose faces had to be totally reconstructed, or the mindless souls that we took to Redskins football games and on fishing trips on the Chesapeake Bay. Not all memories were so brutal. I also remember the wonderful "thank yous" that we received from scores of grateful patients and their families. I have never experienced that type of gratitude since then. I kept telling myself that it was a tough job, but somebody had to *do* it!

Scores of military psychiatrists were involved in the treatment of Vietnam survivors. Collins recalls his work with small therapy groups of officers, all of whom had had successful military careers. A few of these officers were alcoholic; some were still suffering from survivors guilt; some felt they were responsible for fratricide. By reliving these events and sharing them with other survivors in the group, they were better able to openly express these emotions. These "critical events debriefings" (Koshes et al. 1995) were as helpful to the patients as to the psychiatrist. Previously, the patients had felt too afraid to speak about their emotional pain. For years, they had suffered in silence but for whatever reasons, they were now ripe for catharsis about their experiences in Vietnam. During the course of these debriefings there was a surfacing of the psychiatrist's repressed emotions about Vietnam, and he was motivated to visit the Vietnam Veterans Memorial to search for the names of classmates.

Stressors of Operation Desert Storm

Operation Desert Storm was the first war in our country's history in which thousands of women, many with young children, were deployed. Separating mothers from their children was one of the responsibilities of a hospital commander, as it was for one of the authors (JLC), who had been assigned to such a post at the Berlin Army Hospital. The responsibilities related to sending military personnel to the combat zone and the rejection of his offer to volunteer for service in Saudi Arabia served to provoke a recurrence of survivors guilt. Other military members assigned to the Berlin Army Hospital also experienced survivors guilt because, being left behind, they were unable to share the dangers or the "glory" of their comrades. To some extent the guilt was diluted as the hospital staff "lost ourselves in our work caring for soldiers and the families," who had been relocated to the Berlin area.

The survivors guilt for Collins was compounded by the fact that his only son was a young officer assigned to a combat unit. He and the others in his unit survived, but the Collins family lived every day wondering if they would ever see their son and his comrades again.

On Being Black in the Military

In the opinion of the authors, being black and in the army is not too difficult if you are an officer or even a higher-ranking noncommissioned officer. Respect goes with rank, and rank goes with ability up to a certain point. Most medical officers reach that point when they attain the possibility of promotion to brigadier general. During Bowen's tenure, 600 colonels were considered for promotion for two general officer positions. The discrimination that Bowen saw in the army between 1967 and 1985 was based less on race and gender than on rank and intelligence. The following incident (from Bowen's memoirs) is illustrative.

In Vietnam, a young black soldier who was in custody for failure to follow orders was brought to my office by a captain of Chinese descent. The soldier, who had seen me on military television, wanted to discuss the lack of drug treatment programs for blacks only. He suggested that such a program would provide an opportunity for blacks to "talk their talk" as they pleased. The soldier, a bright, articulate draftee from Mississippi, commanded

> respect even though he had refused to follow some order and had paid the consequences.
>
> In trying to persuade the army brass that the soldier's idea had merit to it, I came near to wrecking my own career. But, with the support of several white chaplains (all from the South), we were able to set up a meeting where blacks could congregate and display the "centerfold" pictures from *Ebony* rather than from *Playboy*.

After the assassination of Dr. Martin Luther King Jr., the racial tensions that had erupted between blacks and whites stateside soon became evident among segments of the military in Vietnam. The racial conflicts were often compounded by the antiwar sentiments displayed by new recruits—both black and white.

Summary

The foregoing sketches reflect the multiple sets of responsibilities of military psychiatrists as well as the challenges inherent in the fulfillment of these responsibilities. The authors recognize the need for and value of a more comprehensive report of black American psychiatrists in the military and urge the readers to generate interest in garnering information from letters, diaries, videotapes, and interviews with relatives and friends for publication.

In spite of the authors' traumatic experiences of wartime service and personal experiences with prejudice—on the basis of both race and military status—they are proud of their military service and strongly recommend that young medical colleagues consider a career in the military.

References

Collins JC: Physicians on active duty. J Nat Med Assoc 66(4):350–352, 1974
Cornish DT: The Sable Arm. New York, WW Norton, 1966
Greene RE: Black Defenders of America, 1775–1973. Chicago, Johnson Publishing, 1974
Jones F: Disorders of frustration and loneliness. Textbook of Military Medicine—War Psychiatry. Edited by Zajtchuk R. Washington, DC: Office of the Surgeon General, 1995, pp 63–83
Koshes RJ, Young SA, Stokes JW: Debriefing following combat, in Textbook of Military Psychiatry—War Psychiatry. Edited by Zajtchuk R. Washington, DC: Office of the Surgeon General, 1995, pp 271–290

Additional Readings

Artiss E: Human behavior under stress: from combat to social psychiatry. Military Med 128(10):1011–1015, 1963

Black Americans in Defense of Our Nation. Washington, DC, Superintendent of Documents, U.S. Government Printing Office, 1990

Belenky G: Israeli Battle Shock Casualties, 1973–1982. Washington, DC, Division of Neuropsychiatry, Walter Reed Army Institute of Research, 1983

Cowdrey A: United States Army in the Korean War, The Medics' War. Washington, DC, Center of Military History, United States Army, 1987

Jenkins D (ed): Textbook of Military Medicine War Psychiatry. Falls Church, VA, Office of the Surgeon General, 1993

Lee U (ed): U.S. Army in World War II, The Employment of Negro Troops. Office of the Chief, Military History, U.S. Army, Washington, DC, Superintendent of Documents, U.S. Government Printing Office, 1970

McDuff DR, Johnson JL: Classification and characteristics of army stress casualties during Operation Desert Storm. Hosp Community Psychiatry 43:812–815, 1992

Ranson SW: The Normal Battle Reaction: Its Relation to the Pathologic Battle Reaction. Neuropsychiatry in WWII. Overseas, 1949. Washington, DC, U.S. Government Printing Office, 1972

Ritchie C: Washing clothes. A piece of my mind (letter to the editor). JAMA 270(4):435, 1993

PART II

Surveys

CHAPTER 7

Black Psychiatrists and Academia

IRMA J. BLAND, M.D.
BRUCE L. BALLARD, M.D.

The history of black psychiatrists in academia begins with Dr. Solomon Carter Fuller, who was a member of the faculty of Boston University School of Medicine in 1899. After that time, the number of black physicians pursuing psychiatric training grew slowly, as did the numbers of black psychiatrists appointed to faculties outside the predominately black schools.[1]

The 1960s

During the Civil Rights movement of the 1960s, black psychiatrists became increasingly concerned about their small numbers in the overall psychiatric community and their roles within the larger medical community and the world of academia. It was clear that black psychiatrists would have to make every attempt to come to the forefront and become agents of change within academic medicine. Their roles would have to expand to address such issues as the small numbers of black psychiatrists, the paucity of minorities on medical school faculties, and the absence in so many instances of culturally relevant and culturally sensitive curricula.

Black psychiatrists in the late 1960s called attention to the presence and the complexity of major problems in the arenas of psychiatric care of black patients, the dearth of black psychiatrists available, and the lack of attention paid by major psychiatric and medical organizations to these problems. As

---

1. See Chapter 1 for a historical overview of the academic appointments of black psychiatrists.

noted in Chapter 1 of this volume, the Black Psychiatrists of America was organized in part to induce actions by other groups (e.g., the American Psychiatric Association) that would lead to the resolution of these problems. In a series of meetings, concerns were raised about training greater numbers of black psychiatrists to assist in addressing the range of psychiatric problems among black Americans. Clearly, more black psychiatrists were needed to provide direct services, engage in research, and administer programs. Attention was also directed to the need for links to academia. These discussions generated a number of questions: 1) What would be the sources of supply for black medical students? 2) Could those medical students, if available, be attracted to psychiatry as a discipline? 3) If available and interested, would black medical students be welcomed into residencies in psychiatry? 4) Would our psychiatric professional organizations welcome the active participation of and promote the interests of black psychiatrists?

The Recruitment of Black Medical Students

The academic setting is the source of psychiatrists. Before 1960, only 2.2% of all physicians in the United States were black. Seventy-five percent of those black physicians had trained at the two predominantly black medical schools, Howard University College of Medicine in Washington, DC, and Meharry Medical College School of Medicine in Nashville (Petersdorf 1991).

There could not be much hope of increasing the number of black physicians unless the U.S. medical schools with predominantly white student bodies made efforts to train more black physicians. Thus, in the late 1960s other medical schools began efforts to actively recruit underrepresented minority students. These efforts were principally directed at black Americans, but Mexican Americans, mainland Puerto Ricans, and Native American Indians were also woefully underrepresented and were included in minority recruitment initiatives. The Association of American Medical Colleges established a goal that by 1976, at least 10% of first-year medical students in U.S. medical schools would be black students. With the inclusion of the other minority groups mentioned previously, this recruitment goal became 12%, a figure felt at the time to represent the minority population of the United States. Thus, the intent of the recruitment efforts was to reach population parity (Association of American Medical Colleges 1970).

Black American psychiatrists were active in those efforts. James L. Curtis, M.D., psychiatrist and psychoanalyst, was a major figure. He spearheaded minority recruitment efforts at Cornell University Medical College, an institution that, although not having precise historical documentation of the number of black American graduates, appeared to have graduated only about 12 black American physicians since its founding in 1898. (Cornell's first black graduate, in 1915, was Dr. Roscoe C. Giles, who went on to a prominent career as a surgeon [Bishop 1962; Giles 1970]). In 1969, Curtis became an associate dean at Cornell and began the process of moving the institution toward aggressively recruiting underrepresented minority students. At about that time, other colleges also began efforts to recruit minority students to campuses that had previously been almost exclusively white. Many medical practitioners and medical school administrators recognized that successful recruitment efforts depended in part on the inclusion of black Americans in their administrative structures of colleges. The presence of black American physicians at the higher levels of a medical school's administration and faculty was viewed to be evidence of the school's commitment to recruiting minority students.

Dr. Alvin Poussaint became associate dean of students at Harvard Medical School in 1969, a very important development considering Harvard's prestige as a medical school (American Psychiatric Association 1983). That same year, another black American psychiatrist, Dr. James Comer, became an associate dean at Yale University School of Medicine (Who's Who Among Black Americans 1988).

Black American psychiatrists in those administrative positions in academia had to address a multitude of issues. Medical school admissions committees at that time had little experience with black American college students and applicants to medical schools. Those applicants had to overcome numerous obstacles rooted in problems of the inner city or rural public education systems that so many minority students had attended. Other difficulties included negotiating the college climate, active discouragement by many from pursuing their professional aspirations, overt and covert racism, and major financial need. That these students had come to the point of applying to medical school was in and of itself evidence of having overcome remarkable obstacles.

Medical school admissions committees were often baffled as to how to assess this new group of applicants. For many black American applicants, if they were assessed only by the criteria of college grade point averages and standardized test scores, gaining admission to medical schools would be quite difficult. Yet if factors such as motivation, focus, interest in serving others, capacity for leadership, and academic potential in light of disadvantage were assessed, many such students were among the most desirable and needed medical school applicants.

Some admissions committee members were totally unfamiliar with the everyday lives of minority student applicants. Through their roles in medical school administration or on admissions committees, black American psychiatrists, as well as black American faculty in other specialties, had to educate those committees. As medical students, the minority applicants would again have to face many of the same issues they had grappled with previously while also enduring the stresses of a very demanding medical education. Not only did they have to be academically ready, they had to be emotionally ready as well. There was no question that black American psychiatrists, though they did not perform direct clinical examinations, had to assist admissions committees in assessing the strengths and weaknesses of minority applicants.

In the process of working with medical school admissions, black American psychiatrists also had to remain cognizant of the overall "cultural climate" of the particular medical school. To some faculty, black American students would be strangers within the student groups with which they had usually worked. To others, they would be seen as products of affirmative action and hence perceived as not qualified to be among the student body. (Of course, some faculty welcomed diversity in the field of medicine and therefore were quite supportive and served as vigorous advocates of minority recruitment.) There was also a danger that ignorance or unfamiliarity with the societal backgrounds of some minority students would lead to inappropriate selections for medical schools, because the evaluators were so overwhelmed by the adverse environmental issues in an applicant's background that they might fail to see deficits in the cognitive skills necessary to succeed in medical school. The input of black faculty members was also quite important in those assessments.

After minority medical students succeeded in gaining admission to medical schools, black American psychiatrists in faculty and administrative roles had to champion the development of adequate counseling and support systems as those students progressed through medical school. Attrition problems often seemed connected to inadequate attempts to assist students with the pressures created not only by academic demands but also, in a number of medical schools and hospitals, by negative attitudes toward minority students. It was important that the Association of American Medical Colleges (AAMC) lend unrelenting support to efforts to recruit and retain minority students. Although position papers and task forces within the group lent support, many medical school administrators working in minority affairs felt that the AAMC's efforts were insufficient. A small group of minority affairs administrators, predominantly black American, convened a meeting at Howard University during AAMC's annual meeting, which led in 1975 to the founding of a new organization, the National Association of Medical Minority Educators (NAMME). This association has functioned to facilitate recruitment, networking, and advocacy for administrators in the health professions schools.

Recruitment of Black Students Into Psychiatry

Simultaneously, efforts were needed to encourage black American medical students to enter psychiatry and to foster a favorable climate for training during their residency years. A small fellowship program, the Solomon Carter Fuller Fellowship, headed by Dr. Robert Sharpley, was developed to permit a select group of black American psychiatric residents to travel to different U.S. institutions that served large minority populations. This experience permitted those residents to have closer contact with well-known, prominent minority psychiatrists who were directing major programs. The hope was that this experience would inspire the residents toward major leadership positions in the field, including consideration of academic careers that might enhance the psychiatric care of black American patients.

A larger program, established by the American Psychiatric Association/National Institute of Mental Health (APA/NIMH), was developed in 1974. Directed by Dr. Jeanne Spurlock, it was designed to provide minority psychiatric residents exposure to the workings of the American Psychiatric Association (APA) by funding their attendance at APA's fall committee meetings and the annual meeting The group of psychiatric residents included those of Native American Indian, Hispanic, and Asian backgrounds as well as black Americans. These residents would gain exposure to the multiple leadership aspects of the American Psychiatric Association to develop a better sense of issues that this major professional organization addresses and would bring a minority perspective to various committee discussions. It was hoped that these young minority psychiatrists would, through their years of membership in the APA, be active leaders in bringing high-quality, culturally sensitive psychiatric care to patients from minority groups. This fellowship continues to be an activity of the APA, although it now has a different funding source. One of the participants in that fellowship, Dr. Robert T. M. Phillips, succeeded Spurlock as the director of the program; another fellowship recipient is the coauthor (IJB) of this chapter.

It was apparent from the earliest years of the APA/NIMH fellowship that, in assessing the training experiences of psychiatry residents from minority groups, many departments of psychiatry did not include appropriate sociocultural perspectives in their residency training curricula or in the direct supervisory experiences of psychiatry residents. Minority residents reported situations in which they felt a lack of sensitivity to racial and ethnic diversity among psychiatry residents and found themselves in an awkward position as they attempted to correct misinformation and challenge stereotypes.

Training directors were encouraged to add new or additional cross-cultural educational experiences to their residency training programs. This often took the form of specific educational conferences led by grand rounds speakers (guests who speak at regularly scheduled meetings of staff, trainees, and students). The design of those educational programs often stemmed directly from the suggestions of the APA/NIMH fellows. Early on in their careers, the residents were involved in enhancing the academic departments in which they were training. The experiences of those residents again indicated the critical need for more minority psychiatrists in academia.

This need was also apparent in the membership of the American Psychiatric Association, where the Committee of Black Psychiatrists was charged with insuring that the organization's programs did not neglect the problems and needs of black psychiatric patients and black mental health professionals. One of the authors of this chapter (BLB) chaired that committee from 1982 to 1986; even during the decade of the 1980s, when one would have hoped that issues of cultural sensitivity had become more commonplace, insuring inclusion of a minority perspective was never an easy task.

Joining the Medical School Faculty

A true index of the degree of difficulty involved for blacks to become full-time faculty members in U.S. medical schools is the demographic data. In 1978, of 47,140 faculty members in U.S. medical schools, only 802, or 1.7%, were black American. In 1988, when the total number of U.S. medical school faculty had increased to 60,208, the number of black American faculty was 1,103, or 1.8% (Association of American Medical Colleges 1988). In 1993, the total number of U.S. medical school faculty was 73,865, of which 1,533, or 2.0%, were black American. The 1993 data excluded Howard, Meharry, Morehouse, and the Puerto Rico schools, which are predominantly minority schools (Association of American Medical Colleges 1994a).

With regard to psychiatric departments, in 1978 there were 104 black American full-time faculty members out of a total of 5,150 (Association of American Medical Colleges 1988). Thus, black faculty members comprised 2.0% of faculty members. In 1993, of 6,175 full-time faculty members in psychiatry, 190, or 3.0%, were black American (Association of American Medical Colleges 1994a) This represents a 50% increase in the number of black faculty over a 14-year period, but blacks still constitute only a tiny percentage of department of psychiatry faculty members. This is nevertheless above the average overall percentage of black faculty in U.S. medical schools, and it is an indication that departments of psychiatry are recruiting from a small pool of black physicians who are pursuing academic careers.

The question is often raised about the number of black medical students who become interested in pursuing residencies in psychiatry. Data indicating the racial/ethnic distributions within the first postgraduate year (PGY-1) specialties clearly show interest in psychiatry by the 1993 black graduates of U.S. medical schools. Of black graduates that year, 5.1% entered psychiatry, compared with 3.8% of white graduates (Association of American Medical Colleges 1994a). That year, the total number of black graduates of U.S. medical schools was only 6.1%.

These data are important indicators that the possibility exists to expand the number of black psychiatrists in academia through creative outreach to black medical students and psychiatric residents. But many questions have to be answered in terms of the career satisfaction of black psychiatrists in academia, and efforts need to continue to insure that black Americans overcome many of the aforementioned obstacles in the pipeline that extends from entrance into medical school to becoming a part of the academic faculty.

There was a small but continuous increase (1.5%) in the number of black psychiatric residents over the 5-year period between 1989 and 1994. According to the APA Resident Census Data (American Psychiatric Association 1993–1994), blacks represented 6.3% of residents in psychiatric training in the academic year of 1993–1994, as compared to 4.8% in 1989–1990. The number of black psychiatrists in academia, however, lagged far behind. Only 1,334, or 2.6%, of the 51,127 full-time medical faculty were black American. The number of psychiatric faculty was only slightly higher (2.8%). Despite the interests of a number of residents in academic medicine and many programmatic efforts to enhance their preparedness and encourage academia as a career choice, the gains remain rather modest.

We know of black psychiatrists who have labored within academia for decades. They have made substantial contributions in many areas (e.g., research, education and training, administration) and influenced broad policy decisions in mental health. Several among them (although far too few) have reached the pinnacle of their academic careers with major research contributions, national renown, and tenured professorship. Many more, however, with various levels of achievement and contribution have felt that their contributions have gone unrecognized.

Their individual lots vary, but black psychiatrists in academia generally share the same experiences and academic war stories (i.e., lack of institutional support; limited access to a mentoring relationship; a sense of isolation; and the vagaries of institutional racism, sexism, and elitism). The struggles have been many, the psychological burdens great, and the rewards often too few. Many black psychiatrists in academia, like black physicians in medicine generally, have contributed far more than they have received in return. Wilson and Kaczmarek (1993) said it best: these are individuals "whose courage and accomplishments in the face of adversity merit recognition" (p. 1).

What is the experience of black psychiatrists who have chosen to enter academia? How do they define and perceive the contributions that they have made? What have been their hopes, their joys, their struggles, and their disappointments? And what is their final commentary? These are the questions we sought to answer through our survey of black psychiatrists in academia. It was our hope that they would share with us the authentic story of their lives in academia as well as their insights about specific issues for blacks And what has to be done to make academia a better place to be for aspiring young black psychiatrists. It was our intention to give recognition to their contributions and their struggles.

Survey of Black Psychiatrist-Academicians

Methodology

Using APA (1993–94) census data, we identified a total of 1,430 black psychiatrists. This number represents members and nonmembers (including residents in training) of the American Psychiatric Association. It consists of those living in the United States (1,406), Canada (11), and foreign countries (13). Approximately 858–930 (60%–65%) represent practicing psychiatrists.

A questionnaire was used to gather both quantitative and qualitative data. It focused on demographic information, current academic affiliation, and academic rank and academic status. One section was designed to estimate the percentage of time spent in each of five types of activities: research, clinical, administrative, teaching, and other. A Likert scale was used to rate the respondent's level of overall satisfaction with his or her academic career and to rate the impact of a number of factors known to influence academic careers. A narrative section allows for a discussion of these factors and the identification of other issues considered important specifically to blacks in academia.

Responses to the Questionnaire

A total of 123 black psychiatrists responded to the questionnaire. According to our earlier estimates this represents approximately 14.3% percent of the group of practicing black psychiatrists. Seventy three, or 59%, were male and 50, or 41%, were female (Table 7–1). The respondents fell into four groups: those who identified themselves as actively involved in academia (64%), those who had been involved in academia but were now retired (5%), those not involved in academia (22%), and residents in training (7%). A few forms were also returned by others informing us that the identified psychiatrists were recently deceased (2%).

More males (66%) than females (34%) identified themselves as currently active in academia. Males and females were almost equally distributed in the group not involved in academia—52% and 48%, respectively.

Table 7–1 **Respondents to questionnaire categories identified**

	MALES		FEMALES		TOTAL	
	N	(%)	N	(%)	N	(%)
Active in academia	52	(66)	27	(34)	79	(64)
Retired	3	(50)	3	(50)	6	(5)
Not involved	14	(52)	13	(48)	27	(22)
Residents in training	2	(22)	7	(78)	9	(7)
Deceased[a]	2	(100)	0	(0)	2	(2)
Total	73	(59)	50	(41)	123	(100%)

[a] Forms were returned by someone else indicating that these psychiatrists were recently deceased.

Females represented 78% of the residency training group whereas males represented 22%. The residents who responded to the questionnaire indicated a particular interest in academia.

Demographic Profile of Black Psychiatrists Active in Academia

This group was predominantly male—two-thirds compared to one-third females. The largest number (35%) were in their 40s, followed by those in their 30s (27%). Nearly two-thirds of the group graduated from predominantly white American medical schools. Less than one-third graduated from historically black medical schools; of these, 65% graduated from Howard University Medical School and 35% from Meharry Medical College. Eight percent of the total number graduated from foreign medical schools. Included in the foreign medical schools were University of Ibadon, Nigeria; National School of Medicine, Haiti; Autonomous University of Pueblo Medical School, Mexico; and National University of Mexico. The number of black psychiatrists in this group who had been out of medical school for 10–19 years (29%) was equal to those who were 20–29 years postgraduation (28%).

Geographic Location

The largest number of black psychiatrists in academia were located in the southern states (35%). Most of these were concentrated in North Carolina and South Carolina, representing approximately 36% of the total number in the southern region. Georgia, Tennessee, and Maryland followed, representing 11% each. The smallest percentage (1%) was located in the Rocky Mountain states, represented only by Colorado. The southern region was followed by the Midwest (18%) and the Middle Atlantic (15%). There were 9% in the District of Columbia and 3% outside of the United States. Those outside of the United States were in Canada and London, England.

Type of Affiliation

The largest percentage of black psychiatrists in academia were affiliated with predominantly white U.S. medical schools (78%). Fourteen percent were associated with the historically black medical schools. Howard University Medical School represented 36% of this group, Charles R. Drew 27%, and Meharry Medical College and Morehouse Medical School 18% each. Five percent were affiliated with major freestanding psychiatric teaching hospitals or military institutions. Three percent were in foreign institutions. We did not separate from this group those few individuals who were officially on predominantly white U.S. medical school faculties but whose primary assignments were at historically black teaching hospitals.

Academic Status

The largest number of psychiatrists in this group were concentrated at or below the level of assistant professor (46%). Only 22% had attained the level of full professor (Table 7–2). Seventy-five percent of the group were nontenured; only 19% had become tenured. Six percent identified themselves as on a tenure track. In a recent report (American Association of Medical Colleges 1994b), 2.8% of the tenured faculty of departments of psychiatry are black compared to 82.7% who are white. There was an almost equal distribution

Table 7–2 **Academic status**

	N	(%)
Rank		
Instructor	6	(8)
Assistant professor	30	(38)
Associate professor	17	(22)
Professor	17	(22)
Other[a]	9	(11)
Tenure		
Tenured	15	(19)
Not tenured	59	(75)
On tenure track	5	(6)
Time		
Full-time	41	(52)
Part-time	38	(48)
Pay status		
Salaried	45	(57)
Volunteer	34	(43)

[a] Other included advanced fellow, faculty scholar, clinical adjunct, and affiliate faculty.

of full- and part-time faculty (52% and 48%, respectively). A slightly higher percentage of this group were salaried (57%) than were working full-time (52%), suggesting that a small number of the part-time faculty were salaried. Forty-three percent of this group were involved on a volunteer basis.

Primary Focus of Activity

Where are black psychiatrists making their contributions in the academic environment? We asked survey respondents to estimate the percentage of their time spent in each of five types of activities: research, clinical, administrative, teaching, and other. The "other" category was reserved for activities that they considered important but that did not fit into any of the identified or traditional categories. Although only a few in the group specifically identified "other," we suspect that more black psychiatrists are actually engaged in these uncategorized activities. Included among the activities identified as "other" were making policy decisions, working with educators, serving the community as a professional, serving on editorial and other boards, genetic counseling, national consulting, and working with professional organizations.

The psychiatrists in the entire group cited a wide range of involvement in each of the categories. For each category of activity we calculated the mean and the median percentage times. As might have been expected, the largest average percentage time for this group was focused on clinical activities (47%; median, 50%), followed by administrative (25%, median, 10%), research (14%; median, 5%), teaching (13%; median, 10%), and other (1%; median, 0).

Satisfaction With Academic Careers

A Likert scale was used to rate respondents' overall level of career satisfaction from 1 (least satisfied) to 10 (most satisfied). We examined levels of satisfaction as well as average and median scores of satisfaction for the group. For the purposes of analysis, levels of satisfaction were categorized with corresponding scores as follows: very unsatisfied (1–3); unsatisfied (4–5); satisfied (6–7); and very satisfied (8–10). Fifty-four percent of the group were very satisfied with their academic careers, whereas 24% rated themselves as satisfied. Eighteen percent were unsatisfied, and 4% were very unsatisfied.

The average score on the scale from 1–10 for the group was 7.34, or slightly better than satisfied. The median score was 8, or very satisfied.

Outlier Groups

We selected several subgroups from the study group based on certain defined characteristics. We called these "outlier groups" because the defined characteristic made them uniquely different from the rest of the study group. We looked at the gender, academic rank, and tenure status and examined the average satisfaction scores for these outlier groups. These consisted of the tenured group, the research group, the administrative group, and the least satisfied group.

Research Group. The research group consisted of those black psychiatrists active in academia who spent 25% or more of their time engaged in research.[2] The average satisfaction score for the research group was 9, or very satisfied. This group was predominantly male (70%) and made up of full professors (40%). Thirty percent were tenured and 20% were on a tenure track. The average amount of time spent in research for this group was 60%. At least half of this group was represented by persons of national prominence. There were also two faculty scholars. Areas of research included mental health services, child development, school intervention, AIDS/HIV, schizophrenia, movement disorders, psychopharmacology, violence and suicide prevention, and cultural psychiatry.

Administrative Group. This group consisted of those black psychiatrists active in academia who spent 50% or more of their time in administration. The administrative group was very similar to the research group in that it was predominantly male (71%) and made up of full professors (41%); nearly half were either tenured (35%) or on the tenure track (12%). The average satisfaction score for this group was 8. The average percentage time spent in administration for this group was 67%, compared to 7% as the average percentage time spent in research.

Tenured Group. Those psychiatrists in the tenured group were slightly older than the study group as a whole, with an average age of 56.

---

2. In a survey of research activities of faculty in academic departments of medicine, Beaty et al. (1986) found that the median percentage effort in research was 25% for those with M.D. degrees only.

The majority were male (87%) and full professors (87%). Thirteen percent were associate professors. The two females in this group were both full professors. There were several within this group whose research had achieved national prominence. The group consisted of department chairs, distinguished professors, associate deans, national program directors, division directors, hospital directors, and major program chiefs. This was an unusually distinguished group.

Least Satisfied Group

Sixteen psychiatrists rated themselves as unsatisfied or very unsatisfied. Although females represented only 34% of the entire research group, they represented 63% of the least satisfied group. Males represented only 38% of the least satisfied group. The least satisfied group consisted predominantly of assistant professors (56%), with instructors and associate professors at 19% each. The average percentage time doing research for this group was 2%. All of the members of this group were nontenured.

The least satisfied group identified several major areas of dissatisfaction. When we rank ordered those areas that were cited, lack of a research mentor topped the list. This was followed by lack of institutional support (i.e., no time for meaningful academic pursuits because of clinical responsibilities), being out of the loop of academic politics (no opportunities for networking or meaningful collaboration), and lack of diversity (professionally and in the curriculum) or institutional racism. Men in this group more often expressed concerns in the language of "politics" and "institutional racism."

Most and Least Satisfying Aspects of Academia

The responses from the black psychiatrists in our study group regarding most and least satisfying aspects of academia fell into several broad categories. We rank ordered the responses according to the frequency with which they were mentioned.

Teaching ranked number one on the "most satisfying" list. This was followed by mentoring (or being a role model); research; writing (publications); having the opportunity to balance research, teaching, and clinical work; and, lastly, having collegial relationships. Lack of research topped the "least satisfying" list. Racism and sexism ranked number two. This was most often expressed as being "out of the loop," or "pimped" (i.e., being used in a token way to advance research grants or other efforts with no real investment in their involvement or participation). Racism was also experienced as a blatant lack of attention paid to cultural issues as well as the tendency to be expert on, that is, to be boxed into the position of being perceived as the expert on all racial and cultural issues with little or no regard given to the individual's other areas of interest, specialization, or expertise.

Other aspects of academic life that the black psychiatrists in our study group found dissatisfying included academic politics (infighting, bureaucracy) and lack of mentorship. Many found the administrative responsibilities a bother and the workload at times overwhelming. Salary and travel, although complained about, were ranked very low on the list of least satisfying issues.

Factors Influencing Academic Career

A number of factors may serve to either impede or foster one's academic career. We asked the psychiatrists in the study group to rate the impact of these factors on their academic careers as positive, negative, or having no impact. Respondents had the opportunity to list other factors that may not have been mentioned as well as to give narrative comments for further clarification. We examined the percentage of the group rating positive, negative, or no impact for each factor.

Seventy-five percent of the study group felt that their academic preparation had a positive impact on their academic careers. Most of the group perceived themselves to be bright, hardworking, productive individuals who had come from good schools and were prepared for the academic environment. The 10% who rated academic preparation as negative generally commented on feeling they lacked specific research skills (e.g., methodology, statistics, grant writing, etc.).

Although slightly over 50% rated mentoring as having a positive impact on their academic careers, 40% rated it as negative and 8% as having no impact. There were slightly more negative ratings for research opportunities (37%) and institutional support (40%). There was an almost equal distribution on ratings of the impact of writing and publications, and the impact of clinical duties was seen as positive by over 50% of the group. A larger percentage of the group (46%) rated racial issues as having a negative impact on their academic careers, whereas 32% saw no impact and 22% saw a positive impact. Few saw the involvement in professional organizations as having a negative impact (8%); it was seen as either positive (45%) or of no impact (47%). Other positive factors cited included community and family support. Other negative factors included gender, geographic location, isolation, financial support, and administrative duties.

Issues Specific to Black Psychiatrists in Academia

We asked the participants in the study group if there were any issues that they considered to be specific to black psychiatrists in academia. Their responses focused on both problems and needs. As would be expected, there was some overlap with issues that had been previously identified in the list of the least satisfying aspects of academia. The issue of psychological stress as a specific issue for black psychiatrists was more clearly articulated in the responses to this question. In rank order these issues included 1) institutional racism and sexism, 2) lack of mentors/role models, 3) psychological stress, 4) overutilization, 5) need to focus on racial/ethnic cultural issues, 6) large debt loads, and 7) need for research skills training.

Summary

In this chapter we reviewed the history of black psychiatrists in academia and reported the results of a recent survey of a current group of black psychiatrists/academicians. We do not claim that this study group represents all black psychiatrists in academia. It does, however, represent a broad range of black psychiatrists who are active in academia, in both full- and part-time capacities, throughout the United States, in Canada, and in England.

Those psychiatrists who responded to the questionnaire appeared eager to share their experiences. Comments were candid and emotionally charged regarding previous experiences, struggles, successes, and regrets. The most successful within this group also had poignant stories to tell. Some sent personal notes applauding the study, expressing interest and curiosity about the results, and offering further comments or assistance. Although not asked to do so, many sent copies of their curriculum vitae, articles of their original research, business cards, newspaper articles written about them, and copies of brochures of programs they had been responsible for developing. One child psychiatrist shared with us a copy of his local newspaper column, "Parenting Q & A," which offers professional advice on parenting issues. It was as if no one had ever asked about or been interested in their work or contributions; perhaps the need to express and give audience to their concerns was long overdue.

The results of this survey reveal some interesting, some expectable, and some disappointing findings. The study group was predominantly male

(66%) and graduated from predominantly white U.S. medical schools (63%). Its members were making their academic contributions in predominantly white medical schools (78%). Significant contributions have been made by members of this group, and some members are of national renown. Despite the substantial achievements of many, however, overall only 22% of black psychiatrists in academia represented by this group had attained the level of full professor. Seventy-five percent of the group were not tenured or on a tenure track. There was a large percentage of volunteer faculty, suggesting a significant commitment to education and training.

Teaching ranked number one on the list of most satisfying aspects of academia, followed by mentoring and research. The majority of the psychiatrists in the study group entered academia because they enjoyed teaching. In their mentoring roles there was a sense of "imparting knowledge," "influencing thought," and watching the growth and development of students. In addition to having a direct influence on the professional lives of students, this group took pleasure in the process of formulating and exploring their own ideas and generating new knowledge through research and in writing and publications. There was also a particular emphasis on impacting broad social policy and translating their knowledge to apply "in the real world."

The level of satisfaction with their academic careers varied among the members of this study group along predictable parameters. The average satisfaction score for the group was 7.34, slightly better than satisfied, with a median score of 8, or very satisfied. Higher levels of satisfaction were seen for those who had a primary focus in research or administration or were tenured. Broomes et al. (1992), in a survey of two groups of black psychiatrists, suggested that administration generally tended to be a favored primary focus area for a significant percentage of black psychiatrists.

The lack of research was on top of the list as a reason for dissatisfaction. Approximately 40% of the group considered this to have had a negative impact on their academic careers. Black psychiatrists measure themselves by the same standards in academia as psychiatrists in general. The formulation and conduct of research is equated with success in academia whereas other important contributions, including teaching, are relegated to second-class status. Several issues were identified as contributing to the lack of research. These included lack of a research mentor, lack of research skills (particularly grant writing), as well as lack of protected time, funding, resources, or simply the opportunity for research.

The least satisfied fell out along gender lines, with women concentrated at the lower ranks, feeling impeded in their academic advancement and dissatisfied with their academic careers. Black women psychiatrists, like women psychiatrists in general, face additional issues that undermine their efforts, impede their academic advancement, and lead to feelings of dissatisfaction with their academic careers. The academic politics and disincentives affecting the career choices for women in psychiatry have been described previously in the literature. (Nadelson et al. 1986; Robinowitz et al. 1981).

Regardless of age, academic rank, level of satisfaction, or overall success in their academic careers, most of the participants considered institutional racism and sexism a major issue that black psychiatrists still had to contend with. This was defined as "denial of difference," with lack of attention given to racial and ethnic cultural issues in the curriculum and in research and clinical situations; being "used" only because they are black (i.e., being "pimped"); being pigeonholed into dealing only with racial and ethnic cultural issues; lack of institutional support (especially for nonmainstream areas of research); and being "out of the network" (an obstacle to attaining tenure and promotions and a factor responsible for the "glass ceiling").

Lack of access to mentoring and role models also remains a core issue for black psychiatrists in academia. Some psychiatrists had either established relationships with a mentor locally, created a national network of mentors, or participated in a structured mentoring program. Many more lacked mentoring relationships and saw this as a specific issue that impeded their advancement in academia.

The sense of being under scrutiny, with unrealistic pressures to perform; the need to prove oneself in order to gain credibility; feelings of isolation from self, others, and community; and struggles regarding personal choices and prestige lead to substantial psychological stress for black psychiatrists. Additionally, they often report being the only black psychiatrist in their setting and are therefore overutilized with a myriad of responsibilities, expectations, and obligations. This may include being expected to serve the community, manage crisis, mentor, and serve as a role model for minority students. Outside the immediate setting there may also be the sense of obligation to make a contribution (large or small) to historically black professional organizations and medical schools. Some members of the group felt that it was the responsibility of black psychiatrists to foster the development of research and clinical programs to address issues of particular significance to black populations. They considered it the responsibility of black psychiatrists to provide the translation and application of psychiatric knowledge to meet community needs.

What this survey revealed in general is that black psychiatrists have entered academia enthusiastically committed and generally feeling academically prepared. Some have created their niche and achieved great success with some support, but mostly through efforts of their own. Others have suffered more intensely the sense of lack of institutional support and have not had access to mentorship to facilitate research opportunities and advancement along the traditionally defined parameters of success. All have more or less struggled with what they define as institutional racism and sexism. As a result of this they have borne an additional psychological stress that has siphoned off their energies and perhaps robbed them of the full pleasure of their efforts. It has not, however, robbed them of the capacity to make significant contributions and to make a difference.

References

American Psychiatric Association: Biographical Directory, Washington, DC, American Psychiatric Press, 1983

American Psychiatric Association: Census of Residents, Washington, DC, APA Office of Membership, 1993–94

Association of American Medical Colleges: Faculty Roster System, Women and Minorities on U.S. Medical School Faculties, 1988

Association of American Medical Colleges: Task Force to the Inter-Association Committee on Expanding Educational Opportunities in Medicine for Blacks and Other Minority Students, April, 1970

Association of American Medical Colleges: Minority Students in Medical Education—Facts and Figures VIII, 1994a

Association of American Medical Colleges: U.S. Medical School Faculty, Faculty Roster System, 1994b

Beaty HN, Babbott D, Higgins EJ, et al: Research activities of faculty in academic departments of medicine. Ann Intern Med 104:90–97, 1986

Bishop M: A History of Cornell. Ithaca, NY, Cornell University Press, 1962

Broomes LR, Linn JG, Whitten-Stovall R: Administrative preparation and responsibilities of black psychiatrists in the United States, a survey. BPA Quarterly 19:6–9, 1992

Giles, RC: FACS, FICS, 1890–1970. J Natl Med Assn 6:254–256, 1970

Nadelson CC, Coffey R, Gean N: Incentives and disincentives influencing the choice of clinical psychiatric research careers by women, in Clinical Research Concerns in Psychiatry. Edited by Pincus HA, Pardes H. Washington, DC, American Psychiatric Press, 1986, pp 81–97

Petersdorf RG: Not a choice, an obligation. Presented at the annual meeting of the Association of American Medical Colleges, Washington, DC, Nov 10, 1991

Robinowitz CB, Nadelson CC, Notman MT: Women in academic psychiatry: Politics and progress. Am J Psychiatry 138:1347–1362, 1981

Wilson DE, Kaczmarek JM: The history of African-American physicians and medicine in the United States. Journal of the Association for Academic Minority Physicians 4:93–98, 1993

Who's Who Among Black Americans. 5th Edition. Lake Forest, Educational Communications, Inc., 1988

CHAPTER 8

Child and Adolescent Psychiatrists

DONNA M. NORRIS, M.D.
JOSHUA W. CALHOUN, M.D.
RUTH L. FULLER, M.D.
HARRY H. WRIGHT, M.D., M.B.A.

The authors, who completed child psychiatry training during a wide range of years (1965–1987) and who practiced in different geographical areas (DMN in Boston, JWC in St. Louis, RLF in New York and Denver, and HHW in Columbia, South Carolina), hold the view that our experiences reflect those of a very large number, if not all, of the 60 black child psychiatrists that we have identified. We were aware of the history of a number who had preceded us and note here, in a summarized form, several—all of whom have been role models for many.

Our Predecessors

The contributions of James Bell, Margaret Morgan Lawrence, Mae McMillan, and Jeanne Spurlock warrant attention in any discussion of the "first generation" of black child and adolescent psychiatrists. After formal training in pediatrics and a brief academic career at Meharry Medical College, Lawrence pursued psychiatric training (general psychiatry at Columbia and child psychiatry at the New York Psychiatric Institute). In 1963 she organized developmental psychiatry services for infants, young children, and their families at Harlem Hospital Medical Center. This experience served as a frame of reference for her book *Inner City Families: Development of Ego Under Stress* (Lawrence 1975). A moving account of her life and work is recorded in her biography, *Balm in Gilead: Journey of a Healer* (Lightfoot

1988). Bell completed child psychiatry training at the Menninger Foundation in 1957 and then went on to establish a career in working with delinquent adolescents in a residential setting, the Berkshire Center and Services for Youth. To the authors' knowledge, Mae McMillan is the only black American child psychiatrist to have received some of her training at the Hempstead Clinic in London. She has received many, many rounds of applause for her mentorship and supervision of trainees at Baylor University College of Medicine, where she completed her child psychiatry training in 1966. Spurlock completed training in child psychiatry at the Institute for Juvenile Research in 1952. She has held several administrative, academic, and clinical posts (including chairperson, Department of Psychiatry, Meharry Medical College, 1968–1973, and deputy medical director, American Psychiatric Association, 1974–1991).

We are also mindful of Rose Jenkins's contributions as the chief of child and adolescent psychiatry at Martin Luther King Hospital in Los Angeles (1971–1973) and as the chief physician at the Los Angeles County Department of Health Services. Of course, we are aware of and appreciate James Comer's work in the arenas of academe, public education and health, and communications. We know of the positive results of his New Haven–based program for improving the education of low-income, inner-city children (Comer 1993) and of its replication in other cities. We are also knowledgeable of Gloria Johnson Powell's studies of the effects of school desegregation on children (Powell 1973a, 1973b) and of the significant findings (e.g., regional differences, shifts from "dejure segregation to defacto desegregation, and from defacto segregation to uncommitted desegregation" [Powell 1983, p. 469]).

Some of the authors have known, personally or by reputation, senior colleagues who were well known and appreciated within their communities of work. For example, George P. Brown was a trained and practicing pediatrician before pursuing child psychiatry training (1961–1963) at the University of Maryland. William S. Davis Jr. trained in child psychiatry (1952–1953, 1955–1956) at the Brooklyn Juvenile Guidance Center, and later held a staff appointment there, as well as at Catholic Charities Guidance Clinic (medical director from 1959–1972). Leon McKinney trained at the State University of New York Downstate Medical Center and was affiliated with several psychiatric and social service programs (including Harlem Interfaith Community Service) in New York agencies.

In addition to Brown, Davis, and McKinney, others who completed their formal training before 1970 (or very shortly thereafter) and then went on to make significant contributions in academe, administration, clinical care, research, or a combination of these include Milton Adams (Philadelphia); Martin Booth, Carlotta Miles, Averette Parker, Alberta Vallis, and Frances Cress Welsing (Washington, DC); Nancy Durant (Plainfield, New Jersey); Wesley Carter (Richmond, Virginia); Phyllis Harrison-Ross and Don Heacock (New York City); Quinton James (Los Angeles); Leonard Lawrence (San Antonio); Carol Leal (New York, New Orleans, and Baltimore); Nellie Mitchell (Rochester, New York); Dorothea Simmons (Worcester, Massachusetts); Quentin Ted Smith (Cleveland and Atlanta); and William Womack (Seattle).

We acknowledge the pivotal role that Chester Pierce played in child psychiatry. Although not trained in that discipline, he has been a valuable advocate for children as a psychiatric consultant for the Children's Television Workshop and the program *Sesame Street,* which continues to be popular and holds the interest of children across the country.

The Authors' Charge

In developing our accounts of our experiences as trainees and practitioners in child and adolescent psychiatry, we made use of several questions as a frame of reference: 1) Were cultural issues discussed formally in the training program; if so, how? 2) How are cultural issues discussed formally in the program of our current affiliation? 3) What are our current roles in the program of our current affiliation? 4) What is the ethnic/racial composition of the patient population and faculty of our training program and in our current affiliation?

Education and Training: 1960–1980

Beginning in the late 1960s and the 1970s, enrollment of blacks in predominately white medical schools increased significantly. There are many stories to tell about the responses to the new enrollees. Fuller's painful recollections about being part of a very small minority is representative of the experience of many black students. She was one of two obviously black students in the class of 150. Another black student was thought to be Chinese because of her skin tone and the shape of her eyes. In her 4 years of medical school, few of the classmates knew who she was. The sense of being invisible was familiar to each of the authors.

Another common experience was the limited number of individuals in the medical community who were available to provide encouragement and support. One of the authors (RLF) recalled that a black maintenance man was a strong supporter when she was a medical student. He developed a pattern of looking up from the floor he was mopping and saying, "Good morning, little doctor." Shortly before graduation, when she thanked him for his kindness, he responded, "I am so glad to have helped. We're all very proud of you. You're never alone."

Each of the authors, and a sizable percentage of our colleagues, trained at university-based programs that were close to the central city communities. These neighborhoods of people of color primarily were, and still are, in various stages of deterioration. Children from different cultures were represented in our patient populations. Even so, cultural issues were not incorporated into the formal program in any of the authors' training institutions. None of the following volumes were identified or added to a reference list for trainees: *The Black Child—A Parents' Guide* (Harrison-Ross and Wyden 1973), *Black Monday's Children: The Effects of School Desegregation on Southern School Children* (Powell 1973), *Black Child Care* (Comer and Poussaint 1975), *Inner City Families: Development of Ego Under Stress* (Lawrence 1975). The process of ignoring the cultural context in which patients live has proved to fail the patient populations as well as the trainee groups, regardless of their cultural or racial backgrounds. Some professors have frequently avoided any discussion of these issues, whereas others have expressed the view that the cultural and racial aspects were of only minimal importance in relation to a child's other developmental tasks.

In Fuller's training program issues concerning ethnic diversity were addressed in individual supervision, but the didactic curriculum included only occasional material on cultural issues from an international perspective. Diversity as a part of life and as a required subject for trainees was not included. Wright, who trained in South Carolina, learned about cultural issues "on my own." His interest in African American anthropology and the history of South Carolina, which developed in his college years, provided a sound frame of reference. Two of us (JWC and DMN) trained in Boston at a time when many of the city's residents were strongly protesting the forced-busing decrees that fostered school integration. We did not have the experiences of supervision that addressed cultural and ethnic issues. When issues such as racial slurs encountered when working with young preoperational children were not processed in supervision, the child's growth in treatment and emotional development often did not proceed. The trainee missed an opportunity to further his or her knowledge of the therapeutic relationship and understanding of the child's development. A case example (JWC) is illustrative.

> During the course of a 2-year treatment with a 5-year-old Puerto Rican male who had been referred because of a disruptive behavior disorder and depression, the patient began referring to the black trainee as "my nigger." The process notes covering those sessions were presented to two different supervisors (both white) for assistance and recommendations. The first supervisor gave no indication of having familiarity with the several issues being presented: the trainee's emotional response to "name calling," possible meanings of the child's communication, and possible therapeutic techniques to use. The material was then presented to another supervisor who suggested that he (the trainee) simply "wait and see" what develops. The trainee soon discovered that the boy also frequently referred to his dark-skinned father as his "nigger," particularly when he felt abandoned by his father and alone. Feelings of abandonment were now resurfacing in the patient as the trainee had begun discussing a decrease in the frequency of appointments (from twice a week to once a week). Over the next few sessions, the treatment focused primarily on the boy's disappointment with male authority figures, including his father.

The trainee clarified his role in the patient's life and what he could expect from him. The word "nigger" was no longer utilized or needed. In addition to the dynamics of the transference relationship as outlined in the case vignette, some discussion of the child's cognitive development is also important in order to understand the development of prejudice in the young child. The trainee must realize that prejudice develops in line with other cognitive developments. Children are taught the values that their families and communities share. Those values may reflect preferences or some of the fixed, false beliefs of prejudice. By the age of two, the influence of these values can be seen (Katz 1976). In this case, this 5-year-old had presented a condensed communication on the subject of skin color to his therapist, "my nigger." The child did not come upon this term on his own. He had been taught. As with all therapeutic work, the meaning of this communication needed to be explored with the patient.

Supervision of this case needed to include ample time for the trainee to acknowledge and explore feelings about skin color and responses to a child who introduces the subject with a highly charged word, "nigger." This work in supervision requires a supportive and trusting relationship between the trainee and supervisor and models a process of case review and self-awareness that the trainee must learn to utilize, when needed, on a regular basis.

Fortunately, for some black trainees a range of supervisors, of diverse racial and ethnic backgrounds and practicing various treatment modalities, has been available. In many instances the trainees have arranged (at the suggestion of an assigned supervisor or self-initiated) supervision with a local black psychiatrist who was not formally affiliated with the training program.

Calhoun noted that same-race role models have been very important to the growth and professional development of black trainees. In some cities senior psychiatrists established networks and arranged for monthly meetings with the trainees (general and child psychiatry). Introductions were made and mentoring relationships were established at the meetings of the National Medical Association (NMA) and the Black Psychiatrists of America (BPA), as well as at the annual meetings of the American Academy of Child and Adolescent Psychiatry (AACAP) and the meetings of the Black Caucus of the American Psychiatric Association.

The training opportunities for the authors have been interesting and varied and impacted significantly by the enthusiasm of the faculty and their ability to keep an open ear to different ideas. Wright described his interest in public health and expanding to administration. His interest in child psychiatry was preceded by his earning a MBA in health care administration at the time of his matriculation at the University of Pennsylvania School of Medicine. Each of the authors, not unlike other child psychiatrists, have had training and practice experiences in other arenas of psychiatry. Other areas of training and practice include psychoanalysis (RLF), forensic psychiatry (DMN), research (HHW), and administration (JWC).

Racist Practices

Although patterns of overt racism declined sharply during the height of the Civil Rights movement, covert institutional racism was and is far from absent. For example, at the end of her child psychiatry training in 1966, Fuller applied for a half-time position at a hospital near her training site. She was told that she did not have enough administrative experience. Later, she learned that a white male peer (who had completed formal training in the same year of her graduation and had no more administrative experience than she) had been hired. She was, however, accepted to fill another half-time position, which required considerably more administrative responsibilities than the job for which she first applied, and involved giving services for a catchment area of 175,000 people. Fourteen months and pages of documentation later, the head of the Department of Psychiatry accepted her resignation as a protest against the assumption that something is better than nothing. Later, her responsibilities were divided among several persons who had been hired.

One of the authors (JWC) recalled that reports of overt racism were rare in training programs during the 1980s; however, covert institutional racism was more likely the norm. Such a pattern was noted in the following situation.

> The position of chief resident in a well-known training program was recognized as being quite prestigious; competition for it was very intense. Never in the history of this program had the position been awarded to a black resident. In 1981 a black female resident was indisputably the best in her group. She had finished first in her medical school class and received outstanding reviews in the residency training program. She was well liked by patients and peers. She was chosen as chief; however, that year the faculty decided to nominate two residents, and a white male was also chosen. In 1982 and subsequent years, the faculty reverted to naming one chief resident. The year 1981 was the only time a black resident was awarded the honor, albeit a shared one.

Diagnostic and Treatment Patterns

The authors agreed that over the years since our training, there have been changes in the patterns of disorders for which children are now referred for treatment as well as a shift in the treatment modalitiesused. Norris recalled from her experiences in the late 1970s that a relatively greater number of minority patients were diagnosed as failure to thrive, abuse, or neglect as compared to those patients of the majority group, who were seen as having a greater range of diagnoses (i.e., psychosomatic disorders, eating disorders, psychosis). Today, these patterns have changed dramatically so that a fuller spectrum of disorders has been noted (i.e., depression, psychosis, and behaviorally disruptive disorders) in both groups. It has been the impression of some child psychiatrists that seclusion and chemical restraint have been used more frequently in some settings with black youth as compared to nonminority youth. One of the authors (DMN) recalled that a black resident received an emergency call from an inpatient unit for medication for an out-of-control youth. When the resident, a black female, arrived on the unit, she observed the identified patient (a black male) interacting appropriately with the unit peer group. The resident perceived the nurse to be surprised to see that she (the resident) was black. After an exchange with the nurse and observation of the patient, the resident determined that medication was not needed. There were no further calls about the situation.

By the 1990s, the training atmosphere had changed significantly, with cost containment a major focus of concern that related to all medical treatment. For the most part, long-term psychotherapy for most patients was out and short-term psychotherapeutic intervention was in. The severe limitation in psychiatric-training funds increased the emphasis on the generation of immediate income-producing services and necessitated modifications in training. Trainees and faculty have been asked to take on more clinical responsibilities. For some trainees this change has meant an increased clinical load in the emergency room. In other instances it has meant that faculty positions have not been filled when vacated by resignation or retirement. Many trainees are moonlighting (in part due to increased financial obligations), which does not allow them ample time for reading and further study. Of course, these changes have had a decided impact on all trainees, regardless of their cultural or ethnic backgrounds.

Research

The contributions of child psychiatrists (i.e., Felton Earls, Linda Freeman, Harry Wright) who are also researchers are outlined in Chapter 9 of this volume.

Practice Patterns and Professional Affiliations

It is noteworthy that most black child psychiatrists have chosen to work in areas that allow a multifocused base to their practice of psychiatry. Many have combined academic interests with private practice, and for some practitioners this has included clinical research. For some, it has been quite comfortable to set up offices in their homes. Others have chosen to locate within the inner-city community, whereas others have gone "downtown" or maintained a mix of locations to better accommodate their patients. A common goal has been a commitment that some part of the practice will be dedicated to working with minority patients.

Fuller's account of "homesteading in Harlem" is reflective of the experiences of other black psychiatrists in different cities.

Having children and returning to three-generational living plus needing two offices for dual-career parents underscored the need for more space than apartment living could support. Moving to the "burbs" was not an option for me. . . . Colleagues (black and white) told me that no one had heard of anyone's having a private practice in psychiatry in Harlem before I did . . . It took 3 years to establish a solid practice, but the area did support a busy part-time practice. I had never intended to move to full-time private practice, so I never tried. Patients continued to be ethnically diverse, with more children and women than men. In terms of the duration of treatment, about half of the practice consisted of consultations to pediatricians and other clinicians, mixed with short-term treatment around foster care/adoption issues and gifted students in conflict about relationships, identity, and/or the next move in their education. The other half of the practice consisted of analysands and other long-term patients.

The issue of race is always present; it may have positive or negative meaning to the patient (and family) and must be addressed. Fuller recalled a situation with a patient who had been referred by a colleague. Upon her arrival at the office, the patient asked to see the doctor. When Fuller identified herself as the doctor, the patient exclaimed, "No, no, no, no way!" Norris recalled a similar experience. The patient accepted the referral, but then queried, "You're Malaysian, right?"

Color differences are frequently discussed right away by children, who point to the differences in skin pigmentation between the therapist and themselves. Fuller noted that children from the majority culture did not seem to engage as readily as their parents, who usually respected the child's choice to continue to work with the therapist.

Black child psychiatrists have become involved in leadership positions within the psychiatric and other medical societies. It should be noted that our involvement has been with the totality of our society, not limited to minority communities. Through her work as a full-time faculty member at the University of Colorado Health Sciences Center, Fuller has worked to develop a curriculum for a continuing seminar on cultural diversity. She has served as a consultant to the Sickle Cell Center at Children's Hospital in Denver and the JFK Center for Developmental Disabilities. A sizable percentage of her "organization time" has been given to committee work of the American Psychoanalytic Association and the state of Colorado. In addition to private practice and a clinical faculty appointment at Children's Hospital, Norris has served as the medical director of a multidisciplinary mental health clinic. She has also served as a member of the Massachusetts State Advisory Committee for Mental Health and Retardation and as a member of that state's board of registration in medicine. The greater percentage of her organization time has been given to programs of the American Psychiatric Association (APA), including her electionto the Assembly of District Branches. In addition to maintaining an active private practice, Calhoun heads child and adolescent services at St. John's Mercy Medical Center in St. Louis and is a member of the clinical faculty at St. Louis University College of Medicine. Calhoun has been an active contributor to APA programs, including committee work. Wright's work in the academic arena has earned him promotion to the rank of professor at University of South Carolina School of Medicine. He notes that his research and scholarly production has been both diverse and extensive, but centers on three themes: young children, cultural issues, and management. His organizational activities have been focused on APA programs and those of the American Academy of Child and Adolescent Psychiatry (AACAP).

Each of the authors has been an active advocate for the inclusion of culturally relevant issues in psychiatric curricula. Wright coordinates these efforts at the University of South Carolina, where there has been a shift from specific lectures on ethnic groups and cultural issues to the incorporation of ethnic and cultural issues in nearly all of the didactic and clinical training. Three factors have been operative in this transition, which has been relatively smooth: 1) changes in the physical environment of the service programs, which made them more inviting for ethnically diverse populations; 2) an increase in the number of non-Europeans in the patient population; 3) increased cultural competence of the staff.

A Limited Supply

The reservoir of black child psychiatrists in this country is far below the need. Unlike other subspecialists in medicine, their voices are needed beyond the hospitals and clinics and into schools, foster care agencies, and the juvenile justice system. To ensure the growth of future generations of well-trained child psychiatrists, we must continue to develop and maintain networks of support and to recruit black faculty into key training programs.

Future Opportunities

As we move beyond the year 2000, child psychiatrists will confront significant challenges and unique opportunities. As systems of care undergo dramatic change, black child psychiatrists will need to assume positions of leadership in the subspecialty. Access to and the delivery of psychiatric treatment in America will be profoundly different from that of past generations. The racial and ethnic composition of the United States will also change over the next several years. With the likely adoption of some form of health care reform, child psychiatrists will have the opportunity to treat populations that have been excluded, mainly minorities and the poor. The relevance and importance of culture on development will become more apparent. Clinicians will have to broaden their assessment, diagnostic, and treatment approaches to include cultural differences, poverty, discrimination, and acculturation issues. In addition to the traditional treatment approaches, a broad array of treatment options will be available and will perhaps be more appropriate for children and adolescents of some ethnic groups in our diverse populations. Definitions of care, systems of care, and those providing the treatment and services will broaden.

To impact the health care systems of the future, black child psychiatrists will need to assume leadership positions in education and research. Opportunities for research and mentorships need to begin by the time an individual enters medical school. In 1991, the American Academy of Child and Adolescent Psychiatry's Office of Research established the James Comer Minority Research Fellowship for medical students. The fellowship encourages outstanding minority medical students to pursue careers in child and adolescent psychiatric research and provides early exposure to state-of-the-art research on child and adolescent mental disorders.

As health systems begin to reform, child psychiatric services will need to be both accessible and available. To meet these demands, child psychiatrists must understand the economics of the mental health industry and be willing to assume leadership positions in management. Thorough knowledge of the neurosciences will also be required, as well as expertise in cultural differences. Child psychiatrists will be responsible for treating a larger number of children and adolescents, and much of their time will be spent supervising therapists who have less-comprehensive training. Much time will be spent treating those children and adolescents with severe mental illnesses and medical complications. Black child psychiatrists, most of whom will have (as they do now) extensive experience treating children from backgrounds different than their own, must play a pivotal role in these developments. Training programs will need to teach the importance of culture and its relationship to the child's development. Culturally relevant experiences offering exposure and treatment of diverse populations will have to become an integral part of all child psychiatry training programs.

References

Comer JP, Poussaint AF: Black Child Care. New York, Simon & Schuster, 1975

Comer JP: School Power: Implications of an Intervention Project, Revised Edition. New York: Free Press, 1993

Harrison-Ross P, Wyden B: The Black Child—A Parents' Guide. New York, Peter H. Wyden, 1973

Katz P: The acquisition of racial attitudes in children, in Toward the Elimination of Racism. Edited by Katz PA. New York, Pergamon, 1976

Lawrence MM: Young Inner City Families: Development of Ego Under Stress. New York, Behavior Publications, 1975

Lightfoot SL: Balm in Gilead: Journey of a Healer. Reading, MA, Addison-Wesley, 1988Powell GJ: Black Monday's Children: A Study of the Psychological Effects of School Desegregation on Southern School Children. New York: Appleton-Century-Croft, 1973a

Powell GJ: The self-concept of white and black children, in Racism and Mental Health. Edited by Willie CV, Kramer BM, Brown BS. Pittsburgh: University of Pittsburgh Press, 1973b, pp 299–318

Powell GJ: School desegregation: the psychological, social, and educational implications, in The Psychosocial Development of Minority Group Children. Edited by Powell GJ, Yamamoto J, Romero A, Morales A. New York: Brunner/Mazel, 1983, pp 473–483

CHAPTER 9

Black Psychiatric Researchers

F. M. Baker, M.D., M.P.H.
Tana A. Grady-Weliky, M.D.

Background and Historical Perspectives

This chapter will describe a group of present-day black psychiatric researchers who were surveyed about their formal research training, current research interests, and active projects. A paucity of black psychiatrists are currently engaged in either academic or full-time research careers. Frequently, black psychiatrists do not consider research as part of their careers because of the negative historical perception of research within the black community (e.g., the Tuskegee syphilis experiment [Roy 1995; Thomas and Quinn 1991]) and a belief that research requires significant additional training beyond residency. Black psychiatrists often spend the majority of their professional careers in predominately black communities and are exposed to the reluctance of patients and their families to participate in research studies.

Another potential contributing factor to the dearth of black academic and research psychiatrists is the limited number of senior black American academic faculty at American medical schools. Only 4% of academic faculty positions in U.S. medical schools are held by underrepresented minorities. Although the majority of these underrepresented minority faculty are black Americans, the total numbers are small (American Association of Medical Colleges 1994). Solomon Carter Fuller, M.D., the first black American psychiatrist, was not only a clinician but a pioneer in medical research as well. He was particularly well known for his neuropathologic studies (Fuller 1907). His perseverance and scholarship have served as a model of excellence for black American psychiatrists who have conducted important research studies during the course of their careers (e.g., Adebimpe 1994; Baker 1984, 1993; Baker et al. 1995a; Bell and Mehta 1980, 1981; Earls 1979,

1985; Griffith 1983; Griffith and Maby 1984; Griffith et al. 1986; Pierce 1968; Pinderhughes 1969, 1970, 1973; Wilkinson and O'Connor 1982; Wilkinson and Spurlock 1986).

The type of research in which black psychiatrists have engaged has been broad based. Early research questions, however, focused on mental disorders in black American communities. These questions included: 1) Were risk factors for specific psychiatric disorders the same among black Americans as among white Americans (Prudhomme 1938, pp. 187–204 and 327–391)? 2) What were the specific outcomes of given treatments for black Americans with major mood and psychotic disorders (Baker et al. 1995a)? 3) To what extent did social class and race affect access, diagnosis, and treatment of psychiatric disorders in black American communities (Adebimpe 1981; Baker 1994; Bell and Mehta 1980, 1981; Butts and Schacter 1968; Cannon and Locke 1977; Comer and Poussaint 1975; Griffith 1983; Harrison and Butts 1970; Hendrin 1969; Jones et al. 1981; Kiev and Anumonye 1976; Pinderhughes 1969, 1970, 1973; Prudhomme and Musto 1973; Spurlock 1973)? and 4) How accurately were black Americans with specific psychiatric symptoms diagnosed in contrast to white Americans with similar symptoms (Adebimpe 1981; Baker et al. 1994, 1995; Bell and Mehta 1980; Bell and Mehta 1981; Coleman and Baker, 1994; Jones and Gray 1986; Jones et al. 1981)? The absence of specific data in the literature encouraged black psychiatrists to systematically address these questions in an effort to establish whether differences existed in these parameters for black Americans with mental disorders. Although they were hesitant about doing research, the importance of finding answers to these questions in order to provide better care to black patients prompted black American psychiatrists to design appropriate research studies. In fact, our sample of current black psychiatric researchers follow in the footsteps of Dr. Fuller as they search for a better understanding of the etiology and treatment of psychiatric illness and serve as role models and mentors to young black psychiatrists in training.

To describe the group of black psychiatrists actively involved in research, we contacted black psychiatrists known to be engaged in research and asked them to identify colleagues who also fit that description. In addition, a broad computer search of the literature was completed, the terms African American or black, mental health, and specific psychiatric disorders. Areas of research in which black psychiatrists were known to have special interest also were incorporated into the search strategy. Authors identified from this search were compared to the established list of black psychiatric investigators. We determined the race, ethnicity, or both of the newly identified psychiatrists by comparing their names with this established list or by contacting professional organizations. A final list of black psychiatrists involved in research was compiled from these sources. The criteria used to define black psychiatric researchers included: 1) being actively engaged in research based on the presence of scientific publications within the preceding 12 months; 2) contributing to the medical literature in peer-reviewed journals; and 3) maintaining a university affiliation. These criteria were established because completion of funded research by physicians in private practice is rare.

Seventeen black psychiatrists who fulfilled these criteria were identified. Although psychiatric residents represent a potential pool of future black psychiatric researchers, they were not included in the data analysis because they did not meet the previously outlined criteria. A semistructured questionnaire with 37 items was mailed to the 17 identified black psychiatrists engaged in research. A cover letter accompanying the survey requested their cooperation in completing the questionnaire and explained that the data would be used to provide an initial description of black American psychiatric researchers.

Results

At the time of publication, 70% (12 of 17; 7M; 4F) of the identified psychiatrists had completed and returned the questionnaire. Two individuals (12%) declined the opportunity to participate and 3 (18%) did not respond. Demographic data (age and gender) of the sample are shown in Table 9–1. There was no statistically significant difference in the number of men and women in the two age groups (Fisher's Exact Test, two-tailed, $P = .5758$). Seventy-five percent of the sample (9 of 12) reported that they completed formal research training. When academic rank (assistant and associate professor compared to full professor) was compared by gender, more black American men were likely to have attained the rank of full professor (45%). The gender difference in academic rank was statistically significant at the .05 level (Fisher's Exact Test, one-tailed.)[1] Seventy-three percent of respondents (8 of 11) did not consider themselves "primarily a researcher." Although all agreed that research was an important component of their work, only 27% (3 of 11) viewed themselves as full-time psychiatric researchers. There was no statistical difference between men and women in their self-identification as research psychiatrists (Fisher's Exact Test, two-tailed, $P = 1.000$).

---

1. A one-tailed test was selected in this case because the sample of black American researchers who were men were older and more likely to have advanced in academic rank.

Table 9–1 **Age and gender composition of the sample of black psychiatric researchers (n=12)**

Age Group	Men		Women		Total	
	N	%	N	%	N	%
30–49	4	33	4	33	8	67
50–69	3	25	1	8	4	33
Totals	7	58	5	42	12	100

Note. Fisher's Exact Test, 2 tailed, p = 0.5758. Not significant.

Of the three self-identified black research psychiatrists, two were men and had a research mentor early in their careers. The one black woman in this category did not have a research mentor early in her career. For the total sample, experience with a research mentor early in their careers was reported by 7 of the 11 respondents (58%). There was no statistically significant difference by gender (Fisher's Exact Test, two-tailed, $P = .5581$).

Most academic institutions emphasize the importance of the publication of papers and successful acquisition of grant funds. Although the weight of these two criteria may vary across institutions, both are important in deliberations and final decisions regarding promotion and tenure. Among responding black psychiatrists, 64% (7 of 11) received funding from one of the components of the National Institutes of Health. Only one of these federally funded investigators was a woman. The difference by gender of black American psychiatrists receiving federal research funding was statistically significant at the $P = .010$ level (Fisher's Exact Test, two-tailed). Although a one-tailed test was considered because of the advanced age, higher academic rank, and increased experience of male black American psychiatrists compared to female, the P values for the one-tailed and two-tailed test ($P = .015$) were the same. These seven black psychiatrists also received non-federal research grants from a variety of sources including state funds, private and charitable foundations, and industry-sponsored (e.g., by a pharmaceutical company) projects (Table 9–2).

The number of published papers by black psychiatric researchers was compared by gender, and there was no statistically significant difference between men and women (Fisher's Exact Test, two-tailed was $P = .2424$). It is important to note that one black American man published 68 articles from his six grants and a second man published 25 papers, representing 18% of the total sample. One woman (8% of the total sample) published 17 papers based upon data from her funded research projects. The research foci of the

Table 9-2 **Funding sources of black research psychiatrists**

Burroughs Wellcome Company
Community Mental Health Center
Institutional Funding—Small Grants for Pilot Studies
MacArthur Foundation
March of Dimes Birth Defect Foundation
National Institute of Alcohol Abuse and Alcoholism
    (RO1 = Investigator Initiated Grant)
National Institute of Mental Health
    (RO1 & Award = Career Development Award)
National Institute of Mental Health Merit Award
    (Award to Senior Career Investigator)
Ronald McDonald Foundation
State Funding
United Way
Veterans' Administration Merit Award

respondents were broad. Specific areas of interest included child psychiatry, immunology, geriatric psychiatry, sleep disorders, violence (homicide and suicide), and cross-cultural issues of diagnosis, specifically, the reliability and quality of screening instruments. Treatment of the autistic child and identification of depression in black children and adults as well as psychiatric symptoms and disorders among AIDS patients were also being studied.

Only one respondent had a black senior research mentor during his career (9% of the total sample). All responding psychiatrists had white senior-level faculty research psychiatrists as mentors during their formal research training (100%; 12 of 12). Forty percent (4 of 10) of responding psychiatrists reported experiencing discrimination during their formal research training. In declining order of frequency, the type of discrimination included 1) limited access to the senior mentor compared to other research trainees ($N = 3$), 2) limited access to laboratory facilities ($N = 2$), and 3) harsher criticism or absence of criticism of the trainees' research proposals ($N = 2$). Specific concerns identified by individual black psychiatric researchers included 1) the senior mentor was involved with doctoral students and master of social work graduate students more than with the blackpsychiatric researcher, 2) the black researcher received minimal institutional support for the grant-writing process, and 3) the black researcher was less likely to be included in social activities of the research group. There was no statistically significant difference between the responses of black men and black women psychiatrists with regard to the experience of discrimination during their formal research training (Fisher's Exact Test, two-tailed $P = .5238$).

Sixty percent of the sample (6 of 10 responding psychiatrists) reported that they experienced discrimination in the process of seeking research funding. In declining order of frequency, the following experiences were described by respondents: 1) initial review groups (IRGs) were not sensitive to concerns involving working with nonwhite populations ($N = 5$), 2) the black psychiatrist's area of research was not identified as a priority area ($N = 3$), 3) the black psychiatric researcher received minimal institutional support for grant writing ($N = 2$); and 4) the black researcher experienced an absence of protected time in which to write grant applications ($N = 1$). There was no statistically significant difference between men and women psychiatrists who completed the questionnaire on their report of discrimination in seeking grant funding (Fisher's Exact Test, two-tailed, $P = 1.000$).

One question on the survey asked, "What, if any, discrimination did you experience seeking promotion?" Eighty-nine percent (8 of 9) of respondents indicated that they experienced discrimination in the promotion process. The items selected, in declining order of frequency, follow: 1) protected time for research was available only with grant funding; without funding, there was no protected time ($N = 6$), 2) no faculty mentor within the department was available to provide information on "how to succeed" at the institution ($N = 4$), 3) the criteria for tenure and promotion were unclear ($N = 3$), 4) there was a lack of research resources for pilot data ($N = 2$), and 5) (written in the "other" category) the black psychiatric researcher received no "early warning" as a first-year faculty member that one needed to publish three papers per year in key journals and obtain R01 funding in order to obtain promotion in that particular department of psychiatry ($N = 1$). There was no statistically significant difference between men and women respondents with regard to the perception of discrimination in the seeking of promotion (Fisher's Exact Test, two-tailed $P = 1.000$).

Significance

There has been little in the medical literature concerning the academic careers of black psychiatrists (see Chapter 7, "Black Psychiatrists and Academia") or career concerns of black women psychiatrists in academic medicine (Baker 1993, pp. 194–201). The small sample size ($N = 12$) of this study limits the generalizability of these data. However, these data provide insight into specific trends regarding career paths of black psychiatrists in America and suggest directions for future research. If the current national figure of 2,000 practicing black psychiatrists, based upon data from the American Psychiatric Association and the Black Psychiatrists of America, is accurate, then only 0.9% (17 of 2,000) of black psychiatrists are involved in academic medicine and engaged in research as part of their career activities. Although there are black academic psychiatrists whom we did not identify or who decided not to be identified in this sample, we believe that no more than 1% of black psychiatrists meet our previously described definition of black psychiatric researcher.

The fact that more men in this sample had attained the rank of full professor may be confounded by the difference in age distribution. If the data in Table 9–1 are further divided into age by decade, 17% of women were between ages 30 and 39 and 17% were between the ages of 40 and 49. In contrast among men 33% were between the ages of 40 and 49 and 17% were between ages 50 and 59. Eight percent of men were between the ages of 60 and 69. Therefore, the men in this sample were older, were more seasoned in their academic careers, and had progressed through the academic ranks as compared to the younger women who were at an earlier point in their academic careers. Our findings suggest that more black American women are completing formal research training and selecting careers in academic medicine. This hypothesis is confirmed by the number of women who are currently participating in or planning to complete advanced training in research fellowship programs.

The specific concerns and barriers identified by the researchers included in this survey may not be significantly different from those of other nonwhite investigators attempting to obtain funding for their original research ideas. Responses from survey participants suggest that black American psychiatrists pursuing research training may differ from white psychiatrists in their ability to engage some senior investigators' interest and support during formal research training. As previously noted, however, the generalizability of this finding is limited in that it is the reported experience of our small sample.

There is a change in the demographics of American psychiatrists over the period of 1980 to 1992, with more women and minorities entering and completing psychiatric residency training (1994 American Psychiatric Association Resident Census—personal communication). It is likely that the resultant decline in the pool of white male psychiatrists will lead to a further decline in those white male psychiatrists selecting careers in research. Because of the narrowing pool of potential research psychiatrists, concern has been escalating about who will generate psychiatric research in the future.

The increasing diversity in the pool of psychiatric residency candidates has the potential to increase the number of minority psychiatrists who pursue research careers. This appears to be becoming a reality. The number of younger black women with research training in this sample reflects this trend.

Only a partial sample of the identified black psychiatric researchers responded to our mailed survey. This subsample has been productive in obtaining grant funding. Research monies obtained varied from small institutional grants of $3,000 to develop pilot data for a national grant to a national grant of $5 million over a 5-year period. A successful academic career is defined, partially, by success in obtaining grant funding from multiple sources and by the number of publications produced. By these criteria, these black psychiatrists are successful in their academic careers.

Future Trends

This chapter was written during a time of change in academic medicine. Currently there is movement toward the establishment of health care reform that is expected to improve access to and the cost-effectiveness of health care without compromising quality. The impact of such health care reform and managed care restructuring of psychiatric services on academic health centers and academic physicians remains uncertain at this time. The potential change in emphasis from medical specialization to primary care, however, may detract from the current focus on the recruitment and training of psychiatric researchers.

Over the past 3 years the number of medical students (white and minority) pursuing specialty training in psychiatry declined somewhat precipitously. This fact provides specific data validating the concern about losing psychiatric researchers in the future. As a result of this concern dialogue has been increasing regarding the source of future psychiatric researchers. The American Psychiatric Association, with funding from the National Institute of Mental Health, developed and has sponsored the Program for Minority Research Training in Psychiatry (PMRTP). This program is specifically designed to facilitate the development of interest in research careers among underrepresented ethnic minority psychiatrists and to pair these young psychiatrists with senior mentors across the country. The PMRTP was initiated by Jeanne Spurlock and Harold Pincus, directors of the American Psychiatric Association's Offices of Minority/National Affairs and Research, respectively. The first graduates of the fellowship are beginning to apply for academic positions, and a significant number are pursuing research careers. Postgraduate programs like the PMRTP should increase the pool of minority researchers in psychiatry.

The results of this survey are encouraging for these psychiatric investigators-in-training, who may have some concerns about the type of support they will receive from senior mentors of a different ethnic background. Although the black psychiatrists who completed the mailed survey reported specific concerns, they indicated that during their research training with white senior scientists they did not generally experience discrimination that prevented them from obtaining the skills necessary to become independent investigators.

Conclusions

We conclude by underscoring the limitations of our data. Determining the scholarly activities of black psychiatrists was confounded by the absence of a database that referenced all published chapters and papers as well as the absence of an organization of black psychiatric researchers. Those familiar with the literature on black Americans and mental illness know that important data have been published as chapters in texts as well as in original manuscripts (Baker 1993; Cannon and Locke 1977; Coner-Edwards and Spurlock 1988; Earls 1979, 1993; Green et al. 1992; Jackson 1991; Kieve and Anumonye 1976; Neighbors 1987, 1990, 1991; Pinderhughes 1973; Prudhomme and Musto 1973; Spurlock 1973; Stewart and Robinson 1992; Thompson and Peebles-Wilkins 1992; Wilkinson 1986; Worthington 1992). The research work completed by black investigators in other disciplines (psychology, nursing, social work) was not focused on in this chapter because of our emphasis on black academic psychiatrists trained in the tradition of Solomon Carter Fuller.

It will be interesting to return to the question of black psychiatric researchers in 2005 to determine whether current trends become realities in the 21st century. It will also be of interest to establish whether the trend toward more women completing formal research training and subsequently entering academic careers results in increasing numbers of senior women faculty in departments of psychiatry across the nation. The next decade should prove to be a very interesting period of transition and growth for medicine in general and for psychiatry in particular, as well as for black psychiatrists interested in academic medicine and its associated research emphasis.

References

Adebimpe VR: Overview: white norms and psychiatric diagnosis of black patients. Am J Psychiatry 138:279–285, 1981

Adebimpe, VR: Race, racism and epidemiologic surveys. Hosp Community Psychiatry 45:27–31, 1994

American Association of Medical Colleges: Annual Report of the American Association of Medical Colleges. Washington DC, American Association of Medical Colleges, 1994

Baker FM: Black suicide attempters in 1980: a preventive focus. Gen Hosp Psychiatry 6:131–137, 1984

Baker FM, Kokmen E, Chandra V, Schoenberg BS: Psychiatric symptoms in cases of clinically diagnosed Alzheimer's disease. Geriatr Psychiatry Neurol 4-71-78, 1991

Baker FM: The black woman academic psychiatrist. Acad Psychiatry 17(4):194–201, 1993

Baker FM: Psychiatric treatment of older African-Americans. Hosp Community Psychiatry. 45: 32–37, 1994

Baker FM, Lavizzo-Mourey R, Jones BE: Acute care of the African-American Elder. J Geriatr Psychiatry Neurol 6:66–71, 1993

Baker FM, Parker DA, Wiley C, et al: Depressive symptoms in African-American medical patients. Int J Geriatr Psychiatry 10:9–14, 1995a

Baker, FM, Velli, SA, Friedman, J, Wiley, C: Screening tests for depression in older black vs. white patients. Am J Geriatric Psychiatry 5:43–51, 1995b

Bell C, Mehta H. The misdiagnosis of black patients with manic depressive illness. J Natl Med Assoc 72:141–145, 1980

Bell C, Mehta H: The misdiagnosis of black patients with manic depressive illness. Second in a series. J Natl Med Assoc 73:101–107, 1981

Butts H, Schachter J: Transference and countertransference in interracial analysis. J Am Psychoanal Assoc 16:792–808, 1968

Cannon M, Locke BL: Being black is detrimental to one's mental health. Myth or reality? Pylon 38:408–428, 1977

Coleman D, Baker FM: Misdiagnosis of schizophrenia among older, black veterans. Nerv Ment Dis 162:527–528, 1944

Comer J, Poussaint AF: Black Child Care. New York, Basic Books, 1975

Coner-Edwards AF, Spurlock J: Black Families in Crisis: The Middle Class. New York: Brunner/Mazel, 1988

Earls FJ: Epidemiology and child psychiatry: Historical and conceptual development. Comp Psychiatry 20:252–259, 1979

Earls FJ: Epidemiology of psychiatric disorders in children and adolescence, in Psychiatry, Vol 3. Edited by Cavenar JO. Philadelphia, PA, JB Lippincott, 1985

Fuller SC: A study of the neurofibrils in dementia paralytica, dementia senilis, chronic alcoholism, cerebral lues and microcephalic idiocy. Am J Insanity (Am J Psychiatry) 63:415–468, 1907

Greene RL, Jackson JS, Neighbors HW: Mental health and help-seeking in Aging in Black America. Edited by Jackson JS, Chatters LM, Taylor RS, Newbury Park, CA, Sage, 1992, pp 185–200

Griffith EEH. The significance of ritual in a church-based healing model. Am J Psychiatry 140:568–572, 1983

Griffith EEH, Bell CC: Recent trends in suicide and homicide among blacks. JAMA 262:2265–2269, 1989

Griffith EEH, Maby GE: Psychological benefits of spiritual Baptist "mourning." Am J Psychiatry 141:769–773, 1984

Griffith EEH, Mahy GE, Young JL: Psychological benefits of spiritual Baptist "mourning." II: an empirical assessment. Am J Psychiatry 143:226–229, 1986

Harrison P, Butts H: White psychiatrists' racism in referral practice to black psychiatrists. J Natl Med Assoc 62:278–282, 1970

Hendin H: Black suicide. Arch Gen Psychiatry 21:407–422, 1969

Jackson JS (ed): Life in Black America. Newbury Park, CA: Sage Press, 1991

Jones BE, Gray BA: Problems in diagnosing schizophrenia and affective disorder among blacks. Hosp Community Psychiatry 37:61–65, 1986

Jones BE, Gray BA, Parson EB: Manic-depressive illness among poor urban blacks. Am J Psychiatry 185:654–657, 1981

Kiev A, Anumonye A: Suicidal behavior in a black ghetto. Int J Ment Health 5:50–59, 1976

Neighbors HW: Improving the mental health of black Americans: lessons from the Community Mental Health Movement. The Milbank Quarterly 65(suppl 2):8–380, 1987

Neighbors HW: The prevention of psychopathology in African-Americans: an epidemiologic perspective. Community Mental Health J 26:167–179, 1990

Neighbors HW: Mental health in Life in Black America. Jackson JS (ed). Newbury Park, CA, Sage, 1991, pp 221–237

Pierce CM: Current status of medical research in Antarctica. Antarctic J, 1968

Pinderhughes C: Understanding black power: processes and proposals. Am J Psychiatry 125:1552–1557, 1969

Pinderhughes C: The universal resolution of ambivalence by paranoia with an example in black and white. Am J Psychiatry 24:597–610, 1970

Pinderhughes CA: Racism and psychotherapy, in Racism and Mental Health. Edited by Willie CV, Kramer BM, Brown BS. Pittsburgh, PA, University of Pittsburgh Press, 1973, pp 61–121

Prudhomme C: The problem of suicide in the American Negro. Psychoanal Rev 25:187–204, 1938

Prudhomme C, Musto DF: Historical perspective on mental health and racism in the United States, in Racism and Mental Health. Edited by Willie CV, Kramer BM, Brown BS. Pittsburgh, PA, University of Pittsburgh Press, 1973, pp. 25–55

Roy, B: The Tuskegee syphilis experiment: biotechnology and the administrative state. J Natl Med Assn 87:56–67, 1995

Spurlock J: Some consequences of racism for children, in Racism and Mental Health. Edited by Willie CV, Kramer BM, Brown BS. Pittsburgh, PA, University of Pittsburgh Press, 1973, pp 147–163

Stewart B, Robinson BH: Role strain and depression in employed married black mothers. ABNF J 3:38–41, 1992

Thomas SB, Quinn SC: The Tuskegee Syphilis Study, 1932 to 1972: implications for HIV education and AIDS risk education programs in the black community. Am J Public Health 81(11):1490–1491, 1991

Thompson MS, Peebles-Wilkins W: The impact of formal, informal, and societal support networks on the psychological well being of black adolescent mothers. Social Work 37:322–328, 1992

Wilkinson CB, O'Connor WA: Human ecology and mental illness. Am J Psychiatry 139:985–990, 1982

Wilkinson CB, Spurlock J: The mental health of black Americans, in Ethnic Psychiatry. Edited by Wilkinson CB. New York, Plenum Medical Book Company, 1986, pp 13–60

Worthington, C: An examination of factors influencing the diagnosis and treatment of black patients in the mental health system. Arch Psychiatr Nursing 6:195–203, 1992

CHAPTER 10

Forensic Psychiatry

LEDRO R. JUSTICE, M.D.

Forensic psychiatry generally refers to those areas of clinical psychiatry that interface psychiatry and the law in courtroom procedures (Maloney 1985), including psychiatric assessment of competency to stand trial, determination of criminal responsibility and mental disability, and competence to contract and to make a will (Appelbaum and Gutheil 1991). In this chapter, the definition of forensic psychiatry also encompasses activities of psychiatrists in correctional settings, including administrative as well as clinical responsibilities.

Clinical and administrative involvement of black psychiatrists in correctional settings is particularly significant considering the large number of blacks who are incarcerated. According to Department of Justice statistics, "Between 1980 and 1993, the latest available data, inmates who were black rose from 46.5% to 50.8%. Relative to the number of residents in the U.S. population, blacks at yearend [sic] 1993 were 7 times more likely than whites to have been incarcerated in a State or Federal prison. An estimated 1,471 blacks per 100,000 black residents and 207 whites per 100,000 white residents were incarcerated in the Nation's prisons on December 31, 1993" (Beck and Gilliard 1995, p. 9). It is postulated that black psychiatrists bring greater understanding of cultural, social, and developmental issues into the evaluation process of black offenders and inmates, and perhaps transcend countertransference and transference issues that are generally considered inherent impediments in the evaluation of black juvenile and adult offenders.

Black psychiatrists have been involved in various aspects of forensic psychiatry in the courtroom and in institutional settings. To gather information about forensic activities of black psychiatrists, 22 black psychiatrists (who were known to work in correctional settings or who are largely involved in noninstitutional forensic practices) were sent questionnaires about their forensic activities. Questions were raised about the nature of their training and forensic experiences, including administration and teaching, adult and juvenile forensic activities, and other aspects of forensic work. Fourteen individuals responded to the questionnaire. Six respondents had training in child and adolescent psychiatry following general psychiatric training.

Forensic Training

Few of the respondents had received formal training in forensic psychiatry. Indeed, training in this subspecialty was generally received during general psychiatric training. For example, the author's training in forensic psychiatry was limited to a rotation at a state psychiatric facility,[1] which had a forensic unit on which were placed the mentally ill who were said to be dangerous. Four other respondents indicated that they had received some forensic training as part of their training in general psychiatry; two of the four had also had forensic training as part of their training in child psychiatry. Each of these five respondents has had extensive training by way of experience. After a decade of practice in child psychiatry, one of the respondents (Rosalyn Inniss) completed a formal forensic program.

Forensic Experience

All of the respondents indicated having a minimum of 10 years of varying degrees of experience in forensic activities. Seven of the respondents also gained experience in juvenile institutional settings. Six reported having positions that provided opportunities to direct some aspect of forensic programs. One respondent has devoted his career to working with delinquent youth in an institutional setting in New York State. For more than a decade, the author was a full-time psychiatrist at a youth training center of the California Youth Authority. One respondent has held a full-time position at a California state prison; another has held several full-time positions at different facilities (John Howard Pavilion maximum-security unit of St. Elizabeths Hospital, Washington, D.C., and Clifton T. Perkins Hospital, Jessup, Maryland) for the mentally ill who have committed serious offenses. Another respondent served as director of forensic services of the Department of Mental Health (Connecticut) and chief executive officer for the Whiting

---

1. Middle Tennessee State Psychiatric Hospital, Murfreesboro, Tennessee.

Forensic Institute, the only maximum-security hospital in Connecticut. In the latter position, this respondent was responsible for the development of programming and practice standards that led to a full three-year accreditation by the Joint Commission on the Accreditation of Healthcare Organizations and recertification in 1993. As the director of the women's inpatient unit at the Michigan Center for Forensic Psychiatry, one of the respondents had the responsibility for developing guidelines and medical criteria for admission of prisoners to a community hospital for psychiatric treatment.

Others who are or were involved in formal administrative positions are or have been responsible for handling jurisdiction over those acquitted of crime by reason of mental disease or defect and determining readiness for parole, dangerousness to others, and need for treatment. Some positions have included responsibility for direct supervision of the work of other psychiatrists, psychologists, counselors, and clerical staff.

For almost all of the respondents, the courtroom frequently provided firsthand interface between psychiatry and the law. Although some focused on malpractice and ethics violations in their practices, there was greater experience in other areas. Expert testimony pertaining to competency to stand trial, mental disability or defect, prediction of dangerousness, not guilty by reason of insanity, amenability for treatment; and criminal responsibility are areas in which these psychiatrists have been involved.

Clinical practice has also provided opportunities for development of forensic skills, and several respondents reported forensic work associated with their clinical practices. One respondent indicated that he has worked extensively with children under the age of 10 and has conducted numerous child-custody evaluations. Others reported extensive experiences in child-custody evaluations and evaluations regarding competency to stand trial, assessment of criminal responsibility, and not guilty by reason of insanity. Adoption has been an area of focus for some, and one respondent has been especially involved with interracial adoptions.

Work Environments of Forensic Psychiatrists

Not infrequently, psychiatrists find working in correctional settings very difficult, not only because of the extensive psychosocial pathology of those incarcerated, but also because of significant differences in professional orientation and philosophy as compared to correctional administrators. What may seem common practice for psychiatrists may be quite suspect to correctional workers and prisoners. This is particularly significant when the psychiatrist is new to correctional environments and unenlightened about correctional subcultures.

The institutional environment, molded by correctional administrators and prisoners, is replete with stress derived from loss of freedom and forced dependence on those incarcerated, near-constant surveillance by guards and security staff, restriction and structure of activity, routine of daily life, and very controlled and reduced contact with family and friends. Stress is also derived from forced conformity to security and prisoner codes of conduct. The former requires adherence to administrative policy, and the latter stipulates conformity with standards defined along gang and racial lines and by other prisoner rules of trust and respect. Requirements for demonstrating strength of character are inescapable and often impede the doctor/patient relationship or the processes of clinical evaluation and treatment.

The pervasive ramifications of stress impact prisoners, correctional administrators, security and custody staff, and psychiatrists. For example, during the course of an annual psychiatric evaluation requested by the parole board, the author explored the sexual history of the examinee, who subsequently reported to a staff member, a peace officer, that questions had been asked regarding sexual experiences. The staff member interpreted such questioning as representing an inappropriate concern on the part of the examiner, which resulted in an administrative investigation. Though the method of conducting a psychiatric evaluation was easily explained, questions suggesting undue familiarity by the examiner generated some exasperation. Fortunately, a more sensitive and clinically informed senior correctional administrator assisted in resolving the situation.

Obviously, this experience provided impetus to learning about correctional subcultures, as one would typically do when moving into other new or unfamiliar environments. A psychologist can gain knowledge about correctional procedures from correctional staff by visiting prisoner living units; learning to review case records with the assistance of a correctional staff member, such as a parole agent; and talking with prisoners. These encounters also provide opportunities to educate staff and prisoners about psychiatric evaluation procedures as well as to learn about gang dynamics and prisoner relationships, institutional race relationships, and correctional staff relationships. Exchange of such information enhances communication between psychiatrists and correctional officers and provides opportunities for understanding law enforcement and judicial philosophy.

Some respondents cited institutional racism as a major factor that influenced their perspective of forensic psychiatry. One noted that some attorneys fail to suspect that the black client may be psychiatrically impaired, thus failing to obtain a psychiatric evaluation for black defendants. The chance of this happening is reportedly increased if the client has no history of psychiatric treatment. Another respondent reported that racial insensitivity is blatant in the correctional system and perpetuated by the lack of social and ethnic awareness and consciousness of both prison administrators and other staff who work there. Black prisoners frequently reported that white guards see black prisoners as more dangerous than white prisoners. Another anecdote recounts a tendency of correctional personnel to fail to classify disordered behavior demonstrated by black prisoners as indicative of mental illness. The story of a black male prisoner who smeared urine and feces on the walls of his cell and ate feces but who was diagnosed as "schizophrenia in remission" is but one example of how disturbed behavior is discounted. One respondent viewed the white guards as threatening in some instances. Black prisoners had reported incidents in which guards had tried to discredit a black psychiatrist in their statements that said the psychiatrist was the "worst doctor" in the facility.

Other respondents reported having been victims of institutionalized racism in their respective places of work. One respondent described multiple instances in which he was passed over for a promotion to clinical director for mental health in a state correctional facility. He cited being told that he did not qualify for the salary that had been agreed upon before his initial appointment, and having less-qualified white individuals appointed as his supervisors on two occasions. A female respondent reported situations that suggested discrimination based on racism, sexism, or both. In one case, a white civil service employee resisted being assigned to her, and in another case two white male social workers sought to undermine her credibility.

One respondent indicated his concern that black defendants might not get competent legal advice from nonblack attorneys or adequate evaluations by nonblack psychiatrists. Another respondent noted that white judges perceive him as being biased toward black defendants and being less competent than white psychiatrists. Another respondent wrote of encountering

> disparate treatment of African Americans and others with different racial identities and cultural backgrounds than the majority population. This has occurred in every conceivable component of the mental health/criminal justice liaison, including the police department with regard to arrests versus referrals to mental health facilities, treatment in jails and prisons . . . I've encountered additional difficulties in the workplace when the caregivers, nursing attendants, technicians, custody personnel are perceived as having lower education and are identified as being more like the acquitee/detainee/patient than the professional staff.

Several respondents noted that many individuals, both professional and nonprofessional, who work in the judicial and correctional systems demonstrate a lack of cultural sensitivity. Although differences in psychiatric diagnosis and treatment of blacks have been reported (Adebimpe 1991; Dunn and Fahy 1990; Flaskerud and Litze 1992; Lloyd and Moodley 1992; Strakowski 1993), the identification of treatable psychiatric disorders that have equitable impact on judicial disposition and rehabilitation has been an issue of particular concern to forensic psychiatrists. These issues have been noted in the literature (APA Task Force Report on Juvenile Justice Issues 1990; Lewis 1991; Norris and Spurlock 1992).

An example of the need for cultural awareness is given in this case:

> A black juvenile prisoner reported to a white mental health clinician that he had been "seeing monsters" in his cell and having the feeling that "spirits" were looking at him while he lay on his bunk. Also, while on his bunk, he felt paralyzed, at times, and could not move. The initial impression was that of schizophrenia. Discussion with the clinician and further exploration with the prisoner revealed much anxiety and depression related to his incarceration and isolation from family. He revealed feelings of being punished because of not being available to take care of the very religious grandmother who had raised him. Supportive psychotherapy (without the use of psychotropic agents) resolved his symptoms.

Teaching Responsibilities

The impact of forces that characterize racism have stressful consequences for black psychiatrists and for others in workplace settings. Aware of these factors, black psychiatrists have assumed the responsibility of challenging such practices within those settings and educating against their perpetuation. All of the respondents have held or currently hold faculty appointments and have been or are active participants in teaching and training programs in medical schools and other institutional settings. Presentations at scientific assemblies, such as the American Psychiatric Association and the American Academy of Psychiatry and the Law, have provided teaching opportunities for several respondents. Publications have also served as a valuable format for teaching. Some of these publications are cited in the list of references at the end of this chapter; others are named in the Appendix, which follows the references.

Summary

Clearly, black psychiatrists have been involved in multiple aspects of forensic psychiatry for at least four decades. Although the number of black psychiatrists has been and remains small, especially in comparison to the need as evidenced by the disproportionate number of incarcerated blacks, they have made significant contributions to American psychiatry. Certainly, there is a need to increase the pool of black forensic psychiatrists and a need for greater involvement of these practitioners in clinical and administrative positions as well as in the arenas of research and academe.

References

Adebimpe VR: Overview: white norms and psychiatric diagnosis of black patients. Am J Psychiatry 138:279–285, 1991

APA Task Force on Juvenile Justice Issues: The psychiatrist and the juvenile justice system. Am J Psychiatry 147:1584–1586, 1990

Appelbaum PS, Gutheil TG: Clinical Handbook of Psychiatry and the Law. Baltimore, MD, Williams & Wilkins, 1992

Beck AJ and Gilliard DK: Prisons in 1994. Bureau of Justice Statistics Bulletin, U.S. Department of Justice, Washington, D.C., August 1995

Dunn J, Fahy TA: Police admissions to a psychiatric hospital: demographic and clinical differences between ethnic groups. Br J Psychiatry 156:373–378, 1990

Flaskerud JH, Litze H: Racial/ethnic identity and amount and type of psychiatric treatment. Am J Psychiatry 143:379–384, 1992

Lewis DO: Conduct disorder, in Child and Adolescent Psychiatry, A Comprehensive Textbook. Edited by Lewis M. Baltimore, MD, Williams & Wilkins, 1991

Lloyd K, Moodley P: Psychotropic medication and ethnicity: inpatient survey, Social Psychiatry Psychiatr Epidemiol 27:95–101, 1992

Maloney MP: A Clinician's Guide to Forensic Psychological Assessment, New York, The Free Press, 1985

Norris DM, Spurlock J: Racial and cultural issues impacting on countertransference, in Countertransference in Psychotherapy with Children and Adolescents. Edited by Brandell J. Northvale, NJ, Jason Aronson, 1992

Strakowski SM, Shelton RC, Kolbrener ML: The effects of race and comorbidity on clinical diagnosis in patients with psychosis. J Clin Psychiatry 54:96–102, 1993

Appendix

A Sampling of Other Publications by Black Forensic Psychiatrists

Davis PC, Dudley RG: Family evaluation and the development of standards for child custody determination. Columbia J Law Social Problems 199:505–515, 1985

Griffith EE: Commentary on Bartholet's where do black children belong? The Politics of Race Matching in Adoption, Reconstruction 1(4): 48–49, 1992

Griffith EE, Duby L: Recent developments in the transracial adoption debate. Bull Am Acad Psychiatry Law 19:39–350, 1991

Griffith EE, Etkin K: Legal rights and involuntary transfer following voluntary admission. Hosp Community Psychiatry 32:319–322, 1981

Griffith, EJ, Griffith EEH: Duty to warn, dangerousness and the right to refuse treatment: problematic concepts for the lawyer and psychiatrist. California West Law Rev 14:241–274, 1978

Griffith EEH, Griffith EJ: Community mental health centers and legal rights. Ann Medico-Psychologiques 137:101–102, 1979

Griffith E, Griffith EJ: The patient's right to protection against self-incrimination during the psychiatric examination. Univ Toledo Law Rev 13:269–298, 1982

Griffith EEH, Griffith EJ: Medication, competency to stand trial and the insanity defense. Yale Psychiatr Q 8:4–12, 1985

Griffith EE, Griffith EJ: Racism, psychological injury, and compensable damages. Hosp Community Psychiatry 37:71–75, 1986

Griffith EEH, Zonana H, Pinsince AF, et al: Institutional responses to inpatients' threats against the president. Hosp Community Psychiatry 39:1166–1171, 1988

Little H, Batey S, Wright HH: Drug use as problem with the law in adolescent inpatients. Corrective Social Psychiatry 31:103–107, 1985

Norko MA, Zonana V, Phillips RTM: Prosecuting assaultive psychiatric patients. Forensic Sciences 37(3):923–931, 1993

Phillips RTM, Caplan C. Administrative and staff problems for psychiatric services in correctional and forensic settings, in Principles and Practices of Forensic Psychiatry: A Complete Textbook. Edited by Rosner R. New York, Chapman & Hall, 1994, pp 388–392

Scales CJ, Phillips RTM, Crysler D: Security aspects of clinical care: one forensic model. J Forensic Psychol 7:49–57, 1989

Young J, Griffith EE: A critical evaluation of coercive persuasion as used in the assessment of cults. Behavioral Sciences Law 10:89–101, 1992

Young JL, Griffith EEH: Experts in church courts: a role not sacred. Bull Am Acad of Psychiatry Law 13:71–75, 1986

Young JL, Griffith EE: Expert testimony in cult-related litigation. Bull Am Acad Psychiatry Law 17:257–267, 1989

Zonana H, Roth L, Griffith EE: Review of the psychiatric examination in the Miroslav Medvid Incident and suggested guidelines for psychiatric evaluations of aliens whose deportment may not be voluntary, in The Miroslav Medvid Incident: Findings, Conclusions and Recommendations. Printed for the Commission on Security and Cooperation in Europe. Washington, DC, U.S. Government Printing Office, 1987, pp 390–414

CHAPTER 11

Black Psychoanalysts

RUTH L. FULLER, M.D
JEANNE SPURLOCK, M.D.
HUGH F. BUTTS, M.D.
HENRY E. EDWARDS, M.D.

Introduction: The Place of Psychoanalysis in Black Psychiatry

Comments about the role of psychoanalysis for black psychiatrists need to be prefaced with comments about the place of psychiatry among black populations in general and black physicians in particular. Historically, the need for black physicians devoted to primary care and selective primary care specialties such as obstetrics and pediatrics has outstripped the supply of such physicians (U.S. Bureau of the Census, Black Population 1790–1978, Table 55; U.S. Bureau of the Census 1995, Table 649; King and Gendel 1995). As members of black communities, the future medical students and physicians from those communities are aware of the need for physicians who provide basic health care to patients. For example, community concerns are more likely to be about the care of those who are pregnant, injured, ill with hypertension and/or diabetes and their complications, living with AIDS, running more virulent courses with some cancers, and generally looking forward to a shorter life span than their white counterparts (U.S. Bureau of the Census 1995, Tables 49, 114, 649). The future physician usually has firsthand experience with the course of these diseases when family members and friends are ill and perhaps die. The future physicians' altruistic feelings are intensified by his or her awareness of the community's need for basic health care. Family and community members do not usually ask young students to consider becoming psychoanalysts or even psychiatrists because 1) familiarity with the fields is more likely limited, and 2) the need for analytic treatment is not the most pressing need. Fuller (1996), among others, reports increasing use of psychiatry by black families. Because traditional approaches to problems for black families *are* more family or group centered than for many white families, black family members often desire to use nontraditional treatment modalities. Utilization of psychiatry also increases when proximity increases accessibility (Klerman 1992; Lewit and Baker 1994). Families have greater familiarity with treatment when a family member, friend, or neighbor has been hospitalized for mental illness. On the other hand, individuals who experience the distress of anxiety and depression, for example, are more likely to take their "troubles" to family members, close friends, "wise ones" in the community, spiritual leaders, and primary care physicians. Often these "troubles" are viewed as either a part of life or signs of needing strengthened spiritual faith.

With this background, the future black psychoanalyst has several issues to consider. The first is that of not pursuing a primary care specialty. Each future black psychoanalyst comes to terms with his or her altruistic feelings and concludes that those feelings will be successfully sublimated within the field of psychiatry as the black psychoanalyst will help increase the numbers of affordable, accessible, culturally relevant prevention and treatment options available to black families (Canino and Spurlock 1994; Fuller 1993). The second issue is how the field of psychoanalysis is perceived. As a treatment modality, the long, expensive process of psychoanalysis is seen as useful, or necessary, by a number of black mental health and other professionals. In the eyes of members of the larger black community, however, the proposal of multiple appointments each week, over a period of years, has not been seen as the treatment of choice. Black families, including professionals, have less total and disposable income as well as a lower net worth than their white counterparts (U.S. Bureau of the Census 1995, Tables 731, 755). The setting of priorities as to the use of more limited monetary resources increases the seriousness of the deliberations. Entwined with the family's economic considerations is the current and multigenerational history of the family's experiences with discrimination in our society. As more than one potential analysand has stated, "White people may have the time and the money [for analysis]. I don't. I have to feel better soon. I have to work, take care of my family, and fight [major and minor encounters with discrimination] *every* day."

A third issue for the future black psychoanalyst is how the field of psychoanalysis is introduced. Training programs vary in their diversity of faculty, residents, and program content. Even in programs in which psychoanalysts maintain prominent positions, it is not likely that a possible future as an analyst is introduced by a black analyst. Modeling as an analyst, recruitment into analysis, and mentoring through analytic training have been and still are the tasks of nonblack analysts (e.g., Viola Bernard, Marion Kenworthy, and David Levy at Columbia). It has not been uncommon for the black analytic candidate to be the only black in his or her class.

The fourth issue relates to the place of the psychoanalyst in the field of psychiatry. Analysts in general, including the black analyst, may or may not have been encouraged to pursue interests and talents related to applied psychoanalysis. In past decades, discouragement was more forceful, particularly when an individual's efforts in the field of psychiatry were presented as being incompatible with being an analyst. One of the authors (RLF) recalled hearing criticisms of those efforts couched in terms such as "contaminating" psychoanalysis when the analyst moved out of the analytic setting, or "wasting" one's time, or not having mastered internal conflicts. Similar observations were cited by several respondents to the questionnaire. Exceptions to this stance have existed and still do exist. Within the field of psychoanalysis, individuals and groups have put forth years of effort aimed at making psychoanalytic theory and practice more inclusive of diversity. Viola W. Bernard was an active advocate during the course of her directorship of the Division of Community and Social Psychiatry at Columbia University (1956–1969) and as the chairperson (1968–1978) of the Committee on Community Psychiatry of the American Psychoanalytic Association. Bernard's efforts on behalf of individual colleagues is documented in the biography of Margaret Morgan Lawrence (S. L. Lightfoot 1988). Since 1968, the American Psychoanalytic Association's Committee on Psychoanalysis, Community and Society has provided a forum in which consultative work in many different community settings is presented to and discussed with other analysts. One goal of this effort has been to define what special skills an analyst brings to the consultation setting. It is within these discussions that the committee members have struggled with the concept of realities and the interplay with internal psychic processes (Committee on Psychoanalysis,Community and Society of the American Psychoanalytic Association 1988). Dr. Elizabeth Davis was an early member of this committee; Dr. Ruth Fuller has continued working with the committee since her appointment in 1978. Other efforts have been carried on by the Association's Committee on Community Psychiatry. The black psychoanalyst has a significant investment in applied psychoanalysis as evidenced by the wide range of efforts reported by the analysts surveyed for this history.

The Questionnaire

Development, Circulation, and Returns

Two of us (HFB and JS) identified 26 black psychoanalysts, trained in the United States, who were known to us. Of the 26 colleagues, 3, Walter

Bradshaw, Charles Prudhomme, and Walter Tardy, were deceased and 2 were ill. One of us (JS) informed 22 colleagues of our project and asked them to complete and return a questionnaire that listed questions about training experiences as well as previous and current professional experiences. Fifteen responded to the request; 7 did not. The illness of 2 likely accounted for their nonresponse. Some information (e.g., the institute at which training took place, years of training) about the 7 nonrespondents and the 3 deceased was known to the authors. Additional information was obtained from 4 of the respondents in follow-up communications (telephone communications [2], correspondence [1], and an interview [1]). Information from one nonrespondent was obtained from correspondence and a lengthy telephone interview. Two respondents had not completed training. One had made a geographical move, and the other has not completed requirements.

In addition to questions related to identification (e.g., name, address, sites and dates of medical and psychoanalytic training), questions were asked about membership and offices held in psychoanalytic associations, significant experiences as a candidate and as an analyst (including those related to discrimination), and transference and countertransference issues (during the course of one's analysis) that were perceived to be related to race.

Summation of Responses to the Questionnaire

The greater number (18) trained in the Northeast; five completed training at one or the other institutes in the Washington, D.C., area. Specific training programs and number of black graduates are identified in Table 11–1.

Only two of the respondents commented specifically on their recruitment into analytic training. For them, the efforts of active recruiters were central. For the greater number of respondents, analytic training highlighted some cogent issues:

1. The future of the black candidate as an analyst and as an analyst for black or white patients.
    Only two respondents made reference to having heard psychoanalysts comment about the "unanalyzability" of blacks. One such refer-

Table 11-1 **Training sites of black psychoanalysts**

INSTITUTE	GRADUATES	
	Females	Males
American Institute for Psychoanalysis		1
Baltimore-Washington Institute for Psychoanalysis		2
Boston Psychoanalytic Institute	1	2
Chicago Institute for Psychoanalysis	2	1
Cleveland Psychoanalytic Institute		1
Columbia University Center for Psychoanalytic Training and Research	2	3
Los Angeles Psychoanalytic Institute		1
New Orleans Psychoanalytic Institute	1	
New York Medical College	1	
New York Psychoanalytic Institute		1
Philadelphia Psychoanalytic Institute		1
Pittsburgh Psychoanalytic Institute	1	
Southern California Psychoanalytic Institute[1]		
State University of New York—Downstate Medical Center, Division of Psychoanalytic Education	1	
Washington Psychoanalytic Institute	1	2
William Alanson White Institute of Psychiatry, Psychoanalysis, and Psychology		1

1. The administrative director indicated that one black psychiatrist had completed training at this institute, but the gender of that graduate was not noted.

ence (reported by a respondent who had completed training in 1955) had to do with the supposed inner hostility of blacks; the other comment (reported by a respondent who had completed training in 1962) pertained to the alleged weaknesses of blacks' ego structure.

2. The match between the black candidate and the white training analyst, including transference and countertransference issues.

Five of the respondents indicated that they were their analysts' first black analysand; five thought so, but were not certain; four were not the first black analysand of their respective analysts.

Three of the 10 candidates indicated that they either were or probably were their analysts' first black analysand and commented on difficulties in having their cultural issues included in the analytic work.

These difficulties ranged from the disregard for cultural issues in the analysis, having to educate the analyst about cultural issues, to cultural issues being interpreted generally as an avoidance of "real" material only.

One respondent (who completed formal training in 1976) identified "the almost universal absence of dealing with the issue of my blackness" in the personal analysis as "clearly a deficit." This experience was in sharp contrast to that of another respondent (who completed training at another institute in 1981), who noted that "many issues were examined from an intrapsychic point of view that had interpersonal/cultural impact. We struggled equally to get an appropriate handle on that material." One example that was offered was distinctly black-related.

Another concern was the analyst's inattention to the black analysand's "first language" in the home and community that might or might not have been the English of the majority population (Butts and Haskins 1973).

3. Class was addressed in some comments. Generally, cultural issues were not included. One exception was noted.

Culture was reported to be emphasized in only one program—Columbia's (at least during the period of teaching by Abraham Kardiner). One respondent referred to his strong objection (which he expressed openly during the training period) to Kardiner's viewpoint (i.e., black psychology is totally determined by the subordinate social caste status of blacks).

4. There were positive comments about supervision and the analysis of cultural issues.

Several respondents noted that cultural issues were taken up in the supervisory sessions that related to the analytic work with patients.

5. The black candidates' match with analysands is not known. Assuming that usually the analysands were white, the processes of the analyses would have followed those described by Schacter and Butts (1968).

Any one analysis may have been catalyzed, impeded, or unaffected by the match of a black analyst with a white analyst.

Note was made of the location of the candidate's office as an influencing factor on the match. One of the respondents had relocated an office from a central location for analysts to an inner-city location with a predominately black population. The institute faculty understood the personal reasons for the move but expressed concern that the new office location was out of the way for potential analysts, who were usually nonblack. Furthermore, the candidate had been informed by black colleagues that there had never been a practice of psychiatry, much less psychoanalysis, in the inner-city location. Over a period of several years, the candidate established a diverse psychiatric and psychoanalytic practice at that location.

The Workplaces

Several respondents made reference to their waning commitment to the practice of psychoanalysis as their attention and concerns were directed to other arenas, including academe, administration, and community psychiatry. The authors' review of the aforementioned responses led them to believe that the respondents continued to make use of psychoanalytic theory in their work.

Efforts that were directed toward providing services for underserved populations are spelled out by Christmas in Chapter 3 of this volume. The involvement of others in various aspects of community psychiatry is outlined in Chapter 1. As clinicians, the respondents presented diverse ways in which they have pursued their talents and the results of their analytic training. None has confined his or her work to psychoanalysis solely.

Five completed subspecialty training in psychiatry—four in child and adolescent psychiatry, one in adolescent psychiatry, one in geriatric psychiatry, and one in community psychiatry. Fifteen of the respondents are or have been actively involved in teaching programs designed for medical students and psychiatry residents. Three of the 15 have also been involved in a training program for analytic candidates.

Some black analysts continued their work in the same setting in which they were located during the period of their psychoanalytic training (i.e., Elizabeth Davis, as head of the Department of Psychiatry at Harlem Hospital Medical Center). Three spent a segment of their respective careers as the head of a medical school's department of psychiatry (i.e., Walter Bradshaw, 1973–1974, and Samuel Bullock, 1974–1977, at Howard University; Jeanne Spurlock, 1968–1973, at Meharry Medical College). As noted previously, most were involved in teaching; most hold or have held academic appointments on the clinical faculty of a medical school in their respective localities. At the time of this writing, two are full-time faculty members (Bruce Ballard at Cornell and Ruth Fuller at the University of Colorado). In addition to formal teaching in classes and supervision, the respondents have been or are involved with education and consultation in various settings in their larger communities and at national and international meetings.

Midcareer interests have directed several respondents to pursue other avenues of practice, as illustrated by Orlando Lightfoot's additional training (1969–1970) and work in geriatric psychiatry and Henry Edward's work in the arena of corrections (since 1978). Most respondents maintained a part-time private practice (utilizing several therapeutic modalities) along with fulfilling other professional responsibilities, as outlined in other chapters of this volume. A few remained in private practice primarily. As of 1995, five of the respondents have retired.

Publications: Reports on the Application of Psychoanalytic Thought

From 1967 though 1994, the respondents have contributed to the literature with papers, chapters, and books. These writings have added to our collective thinking about clinical phenomena, treatment, cultural factors, racism, training, psychoanalytic concepts, psychoanalysis, developmental concepts, and social issues.

Reports on clinical phenomena include the problem with suicide in the American Negro (Prudhomme 1938), the sociopsychiatric treatment of disadvantaged adults (Christmas 1967), measurement of outcomes of methadone maintenance (Curtis and Mike 1978), mental illness in blacks (Davis 1979; Lightfoot 1972), psychiatric interventions with elderly black patients (O. B. Lightfoot 1982), assessment of psychopathology in minorities (Ballard 1989), and mental health issues of women of color (Fuller 1996). Other treatment issues are found in such writings as socialization of dysocial children (Brummit 1978), cultural and ethnic barriers to the efficacy of treatment (Butts 1981), grief (Fuller et al. 1988), dynamic psychotherapy when patient and therapist are black (Edwards 1988), and multiple cultural views of children (Canino and Spurlock 1994).

Conceptualizing data on cultural factors in general and racism in particular has been the focus of a number of authors, including Butts (1971), who focused on the origins of white racism and the implications for professional mental health practice, and Pinderhughes (1971a), who addressed the psychological and physiological origins of racism and other social discrimination. Paranoia and racism was the focus of a publication written by Biassey (1972). Bullock and Houston (1987) called attention to the perceptions of racism by black medical students attending predominately white medical schools.

Many faculty, black and white, have made use of Bradshaw's (1978a, 1978b) publications on supervising and training psychiatric residents to work with black patients. Pinderhughes and Pinderhughes (1982) addressed cultural issues and provided helpful guidelines for the training of psychiatric residents.

A number of social issues have been addressed in the publications of several respondents. The following are illustrative: sociopsychiatic rehabilitation in a black urban ghetto (Christmas 1967), the poverty cycle and paraprofessionals (Davis and Ballard 1974), survival guilt and the Afro-American of achievement (Spurlock 1985), and working mothers (Fuller 1980).

Theoretical concepts have been the focus of several of Pinderhughes's publications (i.e., "Somatic, Psychic, and Social Sequela of Loss," 1971b; Ego Development and Cultural Difference," 1974; "Differential Bonding: Toward a Psychophysiological Theory of Stereotyping," 1979; Differential Bonding From Infancy to International Conflict," 1986).

Some of the writings of several respondents can be categorized under the heading of applied psychoanalysis. Christmas (1974) has made a contribution in her paper on psychoanalysis and community mental health psychiatry, as has Butts (1971) in "Psychoanalysis, the Black Community and Mental Health." Spurlock and Norris (1991) provide another example in their paper on the impact of culture and race on the development of African Americans.

Involvement With Analytic Institutes and Societies: Identification as an Analyst

Twelve of the 16 respondents who had completed training indicated that they were members of the American Psychoanalytic Association; 3 of the 12 were also members of the American Academy of Psychoanalysis. One of the 16 was an active member of the Academy only. One of the 12 had resigned from the American Psychoanalytic Association in 1979 in the 22d year of membership. None of the 16 had been elected to a national office in that association, although one had served on a national component, the Conference on Psychoanalytic Education and Research. One had been elected to a 3-year term, as a trustee, to the American Academy of Psychoanalysis.

Three of the respondents had taught in a psychoanalytic training program (1962–1980, 1972–1988, 1986–1988)—two in the program in which they were trained and one in the current institute of affiliation since 1991. Two of the total number of 26 have been named training analysts.

A Search for Additional Data

A letter requesting information (i.e., number of applicants and graduates, number of accepted applicants who did not complete training or did not matriculate, number of graduates who are now teaching in the institute, number of current trainees) about black American psychoanalysts and candidates was sent to the identified executive at each of the 28 accredited training institutes of the American Psychoanalytic Association. Fifteen responses were received.

One respondent indicated that no information was available because that particular institute did not record information about the race of applicants. Another respondent forwarded some information, although it was stated that records do not note racial identification. Three respondents reported that there has been an absence of black American applicants. Information received from 10 institutes is summarized:

Number of graduates	18
Number accepted but dropped out	5
Number accepted but did not matriculate	3
Number currently teaching in the program	4
Number of current candidates	6

Several respondents reported that black Americans other than psychiatrists are among the graduates of their respective programs. One other black training analyst was identified, bringing the total number of black psychiatrists/training analysts (known to the authors) to three. We know that some of the 18 graduates (identified by the respondents) are included in our original count of 26, so it appears that the total number of black analysts has not increased considerably over the years. One of the authors has had contacts with several candidates who are not included in the aforementioned summary and is aware of their enthusiasm and dedication to their psychoanalytic work.

Future Trends

Although potential black analysts no longer need to come solely from the ranks of black psychiatrists and physicians, some continuing trends are likely to be seen.

The need for medical care of approximately 35 million black citizens of the United States will continue to outstrip the supply of black physicians. For example, from 1910, when the 3,077 black physicians in the country represented 2% of all physicians, through 1970, when 6,106 black physicians still represented 2% of all physicians; through 1994, when an estimated 26,376 black physicians represented 4.2% of all physicians, it is clear that a projected ratio of 75 black physicians per 100,000 of the black population is quite different from the ratio of 263 physicians per 100,000 of the general population (U.S. Bureau of the Census, Black Populations 1790–1978; U.S. Bureau of the Census 1995; Physician Characteristics and Distribution in the U.S., 1995/96). In looking at the field of psychiatry as still the most likely route for future black analysts to enter the field of psychoanalysis, in 1994 the total number of psychiatrists was 37,702 (Physician Characteristics and Distribution in the U.S., 1995/96). However, as of March 1, 1996, the American Psychiatric Association estimates the number of black psychiatrists to be only 1,639 [951 members, 688 nonmembers] (Personal communication on the American Psychiatric Association Membership Database, April 9, 1996).

The potential black analyst/physician's personal weighing of pursuing a primary care medical career will have other influences such as the medical school setting and the school's commitment to increasing the number of primary care physicians.

Even with the current emphasis on training primary care physicians, increasing the small numbers of black psychoanalysts may come about should a greater number of psychoanalysts expand their contacts with the broader communities. The authors have often encountered students and other health care providers who are uninformed or misinformed about psychoanalysis. As noted in a recent report (Committee on Psychoanalysis, Community and Society of the American Psychoanalytic Association 1988), psychoanalysts have the task of presenting to colleagues, and, in turn, future colleagues, how the analyst in the community can have a profound and positive impact on many lives.

References

Ballard BL: Assessment of psychopathology in minorities, in Measuring Mental Illness: Psychometic Assessment for Clinicians. Edited by Wetzler S. Washington, DC, American Psychiatric Press, 1989, pp 259–265

Biassey EL: Paranoia and racism in the United States. J Natl Med Assn 64:353–358, 1972

Bradshaw WH: Supervision in black and white: race as a factor in supervision, in Applied Supervision in Psychotherapy. Edited by Blumfield M. Orlando, FL, Grune & Stratton, 1978a, pp 199–220

Bradshaw WH: Training psychiatrists for working with black in basic residency programs. Am J Psychiatry 135:1520–1524, 1978b

Brummit H: Socialization of dysocial children. Am J Psychoanal 38:31–40, 1978

Bullock SC, Houston E: Perceptions of racism by black medical students attending white medical schools. J Natl Med Assn 79:601–608, 1987

Butts HF: Psychoanalysis, the black community and mental health. Contemp Psychoanal 7:147–152, 1971

Butts HF: Cultural and ethnic barriers to the efficacy of psychiatric treatment, in Barriers to the Efficacy of Psychiatric Treatment. Edited by Kelly WE. Springfield, IL, Charles C Thomas, 1981, pp 26–33

Butts HF, Haskins J: The Psychology of Black Language. New York, Harper and Row, 1973

Canino IA, Spurlock J: Culrurally Diverse Children and Adolescents: Assessment, Diagnosis and Treatment. New York, Guilford, 1994

Christmas JJ: Sociopsychiatric treatment of disadvantaged psychotic adults. Am J Orthopsychiatry 37:93–100, 1967

Christmas JJ: Sociopsychiatric rehabilitation in a black urban ghetto: Conflicts, issues and directions. Am J Orthopsychiatry 39:651–661, 1974

Committee on Psychoanalysis, Community and Society of the American Psychoanalytic Association: Position statement on the psychoanalyst in the community: Observations, clinical theory and technique, and concepts of reality [Unpublished 20 year report to the Board], 1988

Curtis JL, MikeV: Methadone maintenance: measuring treatment outcomes. NY State J Med 78:2175–2182, 1978

Davis EB : Mental illness in blacks: an overview and treatment approaches. J Natl Med Assn 71:1022–1024, 1979

Davis EB, Ballard, BL: The poverty cycle and the paraprofessionals: development and its vicissitudes in the black ghetto. Psychiatr Ann 49:33–35, 1974

Edwards HE: Dynamic psychotherapy when both patient and therapist are black, in Black Families in Crisis: The Middle Class. Edited by Coner-Edwards AF, Spurlock J. New York, Brunner/Mazel, 1988, pp 61–75

Fuller RL: Working mothers, in Women's Progress: Promises and Problems. Edited by Spurlock J, Robinowitz CB. New York, Plenum, 1980, pp 91–108

Fuller RL: Health care must be culturally relevant [column]. Denver Med J, September, 1993, p 5

Fuller RL: Panel presentation: the dimensions of mental health, in Women of Color Working Together; Final Report Nov 2–4, 1944. Edited by Thomann N, Wilson J, Gish C. Denver, CO, U.S. Public Health Service, Region VIII. Printing Bachmann and Associates, Westminister, CO, pp 37–40, 1996

Fuller RL, Geis SB, Rush J: Lovers of AIDS victims: a minority group experience. Death Studies 12:1–7, 1988

King G, Gendel R: A statistical model estimating the number of African-American physicians in the United States. J Natl Med Assoc 87:264–272, 1995

Klerman LV: Nonfinancial barriers to the receipt of medical care. The Future of Children 2:171–185, Winter 1992

Lewit EM, Baker LG: Child indicators: race and ethnicity-changes for childen. The Future of Children 4:134–144, Winter 1994

Lightfoot OB: Personality disrder and outcome in the treatment of late-life depression. J Geriatr Psychiatry 22:147–153, 1972

Lightfoot OB: Psychiatric intervention with blacks; The elderly—a case in point. J Geriatr Psychiatry 15:209–223, 1982

Lightfoot SL: Balm in Gilead: Journey of a Healer. New York, Addison-Wesley, 1988

Pamies RJ, Lawrence LE, Helm EG, et al: The effects of certain student and institutional characteristics on minority medical student specialty choice. J Natl Med Assoc 86:136–140, 1994

Physician Characteristics and Distribution in the U.S., 1995–96 Edition. Chicago, IL, American Medical Association

    Table aa: Federal and Non-federal Physician by Major Categories from 1970–1994

    Figure 2: Trends in the Distribution of Federal and Non-federal Physicians by Specialty for Selected Year 1965–1994

    Page 16: Patient/Physician Ratios

Pinderhughes CA: Psychological and physiological origins of racism and other social discrimination. J Natl Med Assn 63:25–29, 1971a

Pinderhughes CA: Somatic, psychic, and social sequelae of loss. J Am Psychoanal Assn 19:670–696, 1971b

Pinderhughes CA: Ego development and culltural differences. Am J Psychiatry 131:171–175, 1974

Pinderhughes CA: Differential bonding: toward a psychophusiological theory of stereotyping. Am J Psychiatry 136:33–37, 1979

Pinderhughes CA: Differential bonding from infancy to international conflict. Psychoanal Inquiry 6:155–174, 1986

Pinderhughes CA, Pinderhughes EB: Cultural issues in psychiatric residency training: Perspective of the training directors, in Cross-Cultural Psychiatry. Edited by Gaw A. Littleton, MA, John Wright PSG, 1982, pp 247–284

Prudhomme C: The problem of suicide in the American Negro. Psychoanal Rev 25: 187–204, 372–391, 1938

Schacter JS, Butts, HF: Transference and countertransference in interracial analyses. J Am Psychoanal Assn 16:792–808, 1968

Spurlock J: Survival guilt and the Afro-American of achievement. J Natl Med Assn 77:29–32, 1985

Spurlock J, Norris DM: The impact of culture and race on the development of African Ameicans, in American Psycatric Press Review of Psychiatry. Edited by Tasman A, Goldfinger SM. Washington, DC, American Psychiatric Press, 1991, pp 594–607

U.S. Bureau of the Census. The Social and Economic Status of the Black Population in the United States; An Historical View. Current Population Reports, Special Studies Series p-23, No. 80. U.S. Department of Commerce, Economics and Statistical Administration, Bureau of the Census, Washington, DC, 1790–1978

PART III

Personal Reminiscences

CHAPTER **12**

Reflections of a Commissioner of Mental Health and a Head of a Department of Psychiatry

MILDRED MITCHELL-BATEMAN, M.D.

On Being a Commissioner of a State Department of Mental Health

During the 15 years (1962–1977) of my tenure as the Commissioner of Mental Health of the State of West Virginia, it was necessary to be a juggler—to maintain and improve support for patients in the public mental hospitals while trying to obtain new funding and resources for community services. I was the sixth person appointed to this post; my predecessors held the position for very short periods of time—8–18 months. I had the good fortune to be a member of the central office staff, as supervisor of professional services, during the time of the appointment of my immediate predecessor, Charles A. Zeller, M.D. Thus I was very familiar with the operations of the department when I was appointed acting director on July 24, 1962, following Dr. Zeller's sudden death. Furthermore, I was intimately knowledgeable about the history of the Department of Mental Health since it had been in existence only $5\frac{1}{2}$ years when I was appointed director of the department of the newly developing community mental health service on December 18, 1962. This title was changed some years later by legislative action to commissioner.

At the beginning of my tenure significant changes were taking place in the mental health care system nationally. If West Virginia was to be able to benefit from the new resources in federal leadership and financial aid, a number of issues and problems had to be addressed simultaneously and immediately. It was necessary to challenge the traditions of care delivery, although embracing the changing philosophies of care would be more easily accomplished than in those states that had long-standing central departments. Indeed, this was true for the internal operations of the "central office" of the Department of Mental Health. However, the legislated responsibility of the department was to operate five mental hospitals and one institution for mentally retarded children. Each of these institutions had reported directly to a board of public works chaired by the secretary of state. In addition, the community mental health service (consisting of three "guidance" centers) was transferred from the Health Department to the new Mental Health Department.

We began to hammer out the basic philosophy upon which to build the goals and objectives for the mental health program most appropriate to the needs of West Virginians. I was fortunate in being able to recruit a central office staff representative of the core mental health professions who shared my conviction that

1. Patients are to be treated to the best of our ability and then rehabilitated to the best of each patient's ability.
2. The apparent total disability of a person is often not a total disability and therefore we have no right to assume that this state of disability is not reversible, at least in part—with the proper attention.
3. Although treatment and rehabilitation of patients already in the system must be high priority, the Department of Mental Health must also maintain as a primary goal programs that foster mental health and prevent mental disability.
4. Individuals in need of treatment for mental disabilities have the right to be treated as quickly and as close to home as possible, in a setting and manner which preserves their freedom and personal dignity to the maximum degree possible.

Early in my administration, we obtained a technical assistance grant to hold a workshop that was conducted with the assistance of the Department of Health, Education, and Welfare (HEW) regional office. Representatives of the state hospital and community staffs were the primary participants. "Breaking the Disability Cycle" was the theme of the effort. It was our goal to develop ways and means to assail practices that actually contributed to the increases in the institutional populations of severely regressed individuals. A major breakthrough occurred in 1965 with the implementation of a

Volunteers in Service to America (VISTA) project for communities and hospitals. The operation of this project demonstrated the abilities of nonprofessionals to provide valuable supportive services to patients and their families. In addition, these workers were able to stimulate community interest in and concern for the mentally ill and mentally retarded persons.

Other community and hospital programs developed from a similar base. A camping program for hospitalized patients began as a recreational activity, but it provided a significant relearning opportunity for both staff and patients. The Foster Grandparent Program was as significant in benefits for the elderly who elected to be involved as grandparents as it was for the children—the emotionally disturbed, the mentally retarded, and the severely physically handicapped.

Although ongoing efforts were directed toward evaluating the needs of patients and determining the feasibility of developing and implementing community services, it was essential to "keep an eye" on hospital services for those in need of such care. Although aware that a sizable number of elderly persons had been placed in mental hospitals because of a lack of supportive resources in the community, we were also alert to the fact that some could not be accommodated outside the hospital because of the severity of their behavioral impairment. Thus, geriatric units were established at hospitals whenever staff and space were available to begin to address the specific needs of the elderly mentally ill.

Of all the specific programs introduced to try to realize the goals and convictions listed here, perhaps the most controversial was the adoption of the geographic system in the mental hospitals. The geographical system is an organizational pattern that breaks the larger hospital into smaller units in which the patients are from the same home area served by a particular community mental health center. This type of organization allowed the community mental health center staff to relate to a consistent in-hospital staff rather than trying to work with the patients and staff scattered throughout the hospital. The process of establishing smaller hospital units on the same grounds as the large hospital effectively banished the high accumulation of chronic, severely regressed patients, many of whom had better personal attention and stimulus to regain some of the social skills they had lost. Such a drastic move brought many concerns and complaints from some hospital staffs, families, and, of course, their legislators—until the latter began to take their annual tours of the hospitals and could no longer find the large, overcrowded wards of poorly clothed, often naked, severely regressed patients. From this drastic "geographic" change the department acquired two facilities that were developed as regional transitional programs. Some patients who had been hospitalized 30–40 years and who had come to light with the geographic system were moved to the smaller regional units, and from there a high percentage returned to the community. Hospital populations decreased for many reasons other than the geographic system, and I will not describe all of them here. The geographic system was no longer a feasible pattern once hospital populations decreased.

In another category of change it seemed that after the employees of the state hospitals were "deinstitutionalized," we made better progress in treating patients rather than just providing custodial care for them. We began working with the legislature to pay employees a full salary rather than supplementing very meager wages with on-grounds housing and food. We introduced the 8-hour day long before labor laws required it, and orientation became mandatory. The governor called me in one day and said, "I hear you are starting to charge employees for their meals. Senator _____ has had calls from employees at _____ hospital." I reminded the governor that the budget increases to salaries for this purpose had been passed by the legislature and he had signed it. He looked at me a long time and said dryly, "I hope you can make it stick." My reply was, "I will." I did. It was the beginning of improved delineations of the roles of staff—from housekeepers to physicians.

As I noted at the time of my resignation in 1977, my interests and goals have always been concentrated on the treatment programs offered to our patients that in turn are based on the availability of people power.

My resignation statement reflects in part my awareness of the philosophical differences that have served to germinate the splitting of clinical and program issues from those that are related to business and fiscal matters. As noted in another communication (Mitchell-Bateman 1986), a legislator pointed out to me that "the boys out there say you do pretty good, but they have one complaint. You're more interested in getting docs and nurses than fixing up the hospital farms."

In the aforementioned communication (Mitchell-Bateman 1986) I made reference to the fact that I, as a public administrator, found many constituencies of any given program, and each one had its own agenda. Each one formed some opinion about the management of the program as well as the quality of the outcome as compared with that constituency's expectation. Although efforts were made to consider the agenda of each group, it was recognized that, from time to time, it was important to identify priorities and stick with them, especially when communications came from the following: 1) the appointing authority (e.g., the governor), 2) the legislative arm of the state government, 3) the recipients of services (their collaterals and advocates), 4) the peer professional community (advocates and adversaries), and 5) the constituencies that are internal to the organization (e.g., professional and supportive staff of the agency). During my administration I found it helpful to develop communication networks with county clerks, county commissioners, and mental health commissioners throughout the state, and also with sheriffs, juvenile and immediate court judges, and prosecuting attorneys. These networks were developed through meetings with those parties' respective state organizations and by identifying key individuals in each group for ongoing involvement in planning and implementation of programs. When there were challenges to some particular program, this constituent base was often able to defend or support our position. On the other hand, the feedback was valuable in helping us to make constructive adjustments.

In some instances my race and gender appeared to make for problems in dealing with particular situations. The following vignette is illustrative:

> During a meeting of the Senate Finance Committee, I had refused to intercede on behalf of an employee who had made an inappropriate request for a salary raise. Prior to the time of a formal budget hearing, I was advised that this senator would challenge the specific monetary request that I was to make. Indeed, he did; however, his verbal attacks were personal and unrelated to the budget that had been submitted. I interrupted his harangue and, in a loud voice, stated that the budget hearing was not a place to respond to personal charges, all of which, incidentally, were not factual.
>
> Following a period of silence, another senator spoke to the matter. "The doctor has a point. These are not matters for this committee, but she is highly educated and we are plain folk, most of us. She didn't have to cut down our colleague with such big words." The laughter that followed broke the tension, and we were back on track when someone posed a pertinent question.

My interpretation of the event was that the real issue the "attacking" senator was addressing was my refusal of his request. His perception of this incident was that he had been rebuffed by a woman. The issue with the "defending" senator pertained to a man being put down by a woman, not my "big words." It is not clear to me if the actions of either senator also represented some discomfort because I am black, but I sensed my color was more of a problem for the "defending" senator than for the "attacking" senator.

Pierce (1988) has written about the micro- and macroaggressions that black Americans meet with daily. Many, if not most, women in leadership positions experience similar encounters. During my administrations, the senate president at that time was a participant in a symposium designed to assist mental health volunteers in working effectively for passage of legislation. At the end of his formal presentation, the senator added, "Any time your director of mental health is up here, I get ready to vote the way you want. I just hate to see her cry." Fortunately, many in the audience were members of a constituency that we had worked with previously, and they discounted the validity of the comment. Nevertheless, the senator had been able to discredit the quality of my presentation or the merit of the request and implied that my success was due to the fact that he had capitulated—merely to appease a female in distress.

Not all efforts had a successful ending. One of the most disappointing came about when the legislature deleted from the budget a small revolving fund that had been used to assist staff in obtaining additional training. Before the fund was lost, it had assisted persons in pastoral counseling, mental health administration, child psychiatry, nursing, psychology, and social work. Some persons repaid in cash rather than time, so the fund was actually building up a little. But most recipients did return to work in the system and made valuable contributions.

On another occasion we had succeeded, after several years of effort, in getting the legislature to allow a certain proportion of hospital revenues to go into a revolving account for capital improvements at the hospitals. There was only one dissenting vote, but the governor, in the first year of his first term, vetoed the bill. It would be another 8 years before a similar measure was finally passed.

My experiences as State Commissioner of Mental Health did not appear to be substantially different from those of my counterparts in other states. In fact, in many instances, the acceptance of my work by the citizens and professionals was on the whole quite supportive even during the rough times when some legislators or newsperson would take an exposé-type action about hospital conditions. And finally, there were those instances when as the department itself grew, the singleness of purpose was not always present within. This began to be especially troublesome when the chief of administration worked to undercut my authority, creating tremendous conflict in the department. When I requested his resignation, his anticipated support from the governor-elect did not materialize, but considerable damage had already been done to my effectiveness. In retrospect, I again cannot say my gender or my race played any part in this. It is the kind of development that several of my male counterparts had experienced in much shorter periods of tenure than my 15 years.

I have stated previously (Mitchell-Bateman 1986) that when women are aware of the biased notions about women, we are in a better position to ward off a defensive or counteroffensive mode of reaction. Aside from the issues that might have been related to my gender and race, the tasks and responsibilities that I had as commissioner were enormous. It was helpful to me to recall, from time to time, the words of John F. Kennedy: "All this will not be finished in the first 100 days. Nor will it be finished in the first 1,000 days, nor in the life of this administration, nor even perhaps in our lifetime on this planet. But let us begin."

At the time of my departure, there was a new beginning. Then-governor John D. Rockefeller signed a bill that called for the Department of Health to absorb the Department of Mental Health. I left the position (in June 1977) with mixed emotions—sad that we had not yet reached the summit of our goals, but proud to have built, with the help of many individuals, a solid foundation from which a strong mental health program could operate.

On Being the Head of a Department of Psychiatry

July 1, 1977, marked the beginning of my position as head of the Department of Psychiatry at Marshall University School of Medicine in Huntington, West Virginia. Some of my administrative responsibilities were similar to those that I had as commissioner. The school was in its earliest stages of development, with plans to admit the first students in 6 months. Department heads in medicine, pediatrics, family practice, and surgery had been on board from 3 to 12 months or more before my arrival; however, I found an openness and commitment to developing a psychiatric department that would have an integral educational role beginning from day 1 of the first year of medical school. In keeping with the school's goal of preparing primary care physicians who are committed to practicing in rural and small-town areas of the state, the Department of Psychiatry developed clinical experience sites in whatever community psychiatric resources existed. One of the resources was a state mental hospital. Actually, one of the facilities had been under my jurisdiction as Commissioner of Mental Health. I had tried unsuccessfully for years to forge some type of mutually beneficial collaboration between the West Virginia University School of Medicine and another state mental institution. Thus, a part of the attraction for me in joining the Marshall faculty was to see if such a collaboration could be more easily developed working from the university side. Space does not permit a full description of all the experiences I encountered along the way. Suffice it to say that as a result of this collaboration, a clinical director was recruited from private practice who had previously been a state hospital superintendent. He was given a joint appointment in the Department of Psychiatry. I became a consultant at the hospital, at first for a few hours a week, but this moved close to full-time when a unit was assigned to the medical school and students began to spend a significant part of their psychiatric experience in the state hospital. The clinical director, Dr. Roy Edwards, began to chart and guide the clinical services toward meeting the standards of the Joint Commission on Accreditation of Healthcare Organizations. The hospital administrator was a strong implementor and generated financial support from the state. The dean of the school of medicine and my successor as chairman of the academic Department of Psychiatry remained committed so that the hospital was accredited by the Joint Commission, a first for the state of West Virginia.

I have had the pleasure of watching and working with medical students, most of whom start in silent terror but finish their rotation with a wonderful sense of comfort with, and respect for, persons with serious mental illness. Some of them have elected to specialize in psychiatry; most express gratitude for a learning experience that follows them wherever they have gone in their medical careers.

This brings me to a brief statement of another philosophical belief generated by my own psychiatric training and maintained throughout my years as commissioner. I am speaking now of the principle enunciated by Drs. Karl and Will Menninger—"brains before bricks." This really is "conviction number 5," which was a cornerstone for many of our efforts to promote and develop our people power. As I have stated on many occasions, I am well aware that roofs must not leak, paint must not peel, and perhaps some new facilities must be built, but I can never erase from my mind that the way we treat those entrusted to us, the programs we offer them and the staff we acquire to help them are the first and foremost goals to be continually addressed at all levels of a system of mental health care. Whether in the director's or commissioner's office, or the local hospital, or the private-practice group, the individual and his or her constituency must be at the center of any decisions affecting the delivery of services to that individual.

References

Mitchell-Bateman M: The woman psychiatrist in public administration, in Women Physicians in Leadership Roles. Edited by Dickstein L, Nadelson CC. Washington, DC, American Psychiatric Press, 1986, pp 215–218

Pierce CM: Stress in the workplace, in Black Families in Crisis: The Middle Class. Edited by Coner-Edwards AF, Spurlock, J. New York, Brunner/Mazel, 1988, pp 27–34

CHAPTER **13**

Reflections on the Career of a Black Psychiatrist in the Veterans Administration

JAMES E. BAKER, M.D.

The telephone call I received early one morning in January 1961 had a profound influence upon my professional career. The call was from the director of psychiatry service of the Veterans Administration Central Office (VACO). The caller wanted to discuss the possibility of my accepting an offer to be trained to become a chief of staff. At that time, I was a ward psychiatrist at the Veterans Administration Medical Center in Togus, Maine, where I had been assigned in 1956. This hospital, built in 1865, was the first facility for the treatment of veterans of the Union Army.

Introduction to the VAMC System

There is, however, an earlier chapter to my association with the VA system. It began immediately after my junior year at Meharry Medical College when I was selected as an extern at the Topeka State Hospital in Topeka, Kansas. My supervisor encouraged me to attend lectures and seminars for residents who were in training at the Menninger School of Psychiatry. Most of these training sessions were held at the local VA medical center. The knowledge and treatment approach to the mentally ill patients was tremendously different and more therapeutic than my previous concept had been. My attitude and interest in the treatment of those who were psychiatrically ill underwent a major change. Upon returning to Meharry for my senior year of medical school, I had become convinced that psychiatry was the branch of medicine in which I wanted to specialize. Dr. Karl Menninger had encouraged me to pursue this interest.

My rotating internship was at Harlem Hospital in New York City. There, the importance of how psychological factors affect individuals' reasons for seeking hospitalization became increasingly apparent. I was accepted as a resident in psychiatry at the Veterans Administration Medical Center (VAMC) in Topeka beginning July 1, 1953. There were two other black residents in my class and two others in advanced years. Coordination between federal, state, county, city, and private psychiatric programs provided a variety of clinical settings in Topeka. Treatment teams were more than a concept; they were ingrained as the treatment model. It was believed that combining the coordinated skills of various professional disciplines and organizations, as opposed to relying on a solo practice, would be for the greater good of patients. I was in tune with this philosophy to treat patients most effectively.

Throughout the period of my training, a psychiatric resident had to perform as an officer of the day, along with other dutiesthat required the application of general medical knowledge as well as psychiatry. This approach assisted in rounding out an integration of physical and psychological considerations concerning patient care. There was only one supervisor with whom I encountered any difficulties, which I would attribute to racial attitudes. He seemed to delight in making derogatory comments and making assignments that he thought were routine but beyond my abilities. Occasionally, a few patients would make racial slurs. However, I can recall no patient reassigned to another resident because the patient resented the assignment to me. When race-related issues arose during the course of treatment, the patient and I discussed these matters.

On the first morning of my rotation through the outpatient clinic, my first patient, who happened to be a former naval officer, appeared startled when he entered the office. He refused to sit down, then uttered several racial slurs as he proceeded to leave. As he departed he muttered, "What the hell did I do for the VA to assign me to a nigger psychiatrist?" Although he had stated that he would not return, he not only returned the next week but continued to keep his appointments throughout my 6-month assignment. At the time of his last appointment with me, he thanked me for helping him understand so much about himself and wished me the best in my career.

One of the few times I can recall that discrimination worked in my favor was with regard to housing in Topeka. Many of the first-year residents were permitted to live in some old barracks that had been the quarters for the Women's Army Corps (WAC) during World War II. After the first year, these residents were expected to find housing in the Topeka community (the site of the origin of the landmark 1954 lawsuit, *Brown v. Board of Education of Topeka, Kansas*), which was almost impossible for black residents. Therefore, the black residents were allowed to remain in the WAC quarters.

In an effort to attract and retain residents, the VA developed a plan whereby residents would be subsidized for 3 years, with benefits and a salary increase, provided that the residents agree to accept a 2-year assignment to whichever VA medical center was selected for them. I signed this agreement, and upon completion of my training I was assigned to the VAMC in Togus, Maine—a remote place about which I had never heard. In a welcoming letter, I was advised that I would be given a house "on the grounds." Before I began my duty in July 1956, I was informed that I would be the first black psychiatrist to work at this VAMC, and some "uneasiness" existed in the hospital.

The director of psychiatry service may have tuned into my surprised response to his offer (described in the first paragraph of this chapter), and he suggested that I think about the offer before making a decision. He added that he would like to discuss the matter further when he visited the VAMC at Togus 3 weeks later. I pondered the fact that a move from ward psychiatrist to chief of staff seemed to be a giant step. I talked with my supervisor, the chief of staff at Togus; and, of course, with my wife, my closest advisor.

At our meeting the director of psychiatry service informed me that he had received several very favorable reports about my work at Togus over the previous 5 years. He expressed the opinion that a position as chief of staff would give me the opportunity to make broader use of the treatment measures that my team and I were then using on the one ward to which I was assigned. Furthermore, he advised that VACO was interested in psychiatrists who were willing to take leadership responsibility to help implement needed changes in the treatment and rehabilitation of veterans who were mentally ill. At that time psychiatric patients were still under what was called the "3L" program—label the patients, lock them up, and lose the key. At Togus I headed two treatment teams with the direct responsibility of providing treatment and rehabilitation for approximately 200 patients. Although neuropsychiatric medications, chiefly thorazine and reserpine, had been introduced a few years earlier, treatment was largely custodial, with sedations and convulsive therapies. We reclassified all of those patients. Plans were begun to discharge many of them who actually no longer needed to be hospitalized. Some were assigned to return for outpatient follow-up. Each patient who remained received specific assignments geared to their individual needs. Reviews of medications often resulted in their elimination or significant reduction. Patients were assigned to group therapy activities. Participating in activities of daily living and wearing personal clothing rather than institutional attire were insisted upon. Under the direct supervision of a team psychologist, we formed a special group that came to be known as the transitional neuropsychiatric treatment (TNT) unit. The patients in this group were given a special unlocked area on the ward. Each one was trained to keep and take his own noninjectable medications. Each had some work assignment, including the responsibility to help maintain the ward area in tip-top condition. More important, however, was the satisfaction of having paying job assignments either within the hospital or in the community. A portion of the earnings from these jobs was set aside for the patients' reentry into the community. This group of patients were permitted to have passes to leave the hospital grounds without being accompanied by a relative or staff member when not on duty. Activities would be planned, such as trips to see professional baseball games in Boston followed by dinner at a fancy restaurant. These changes, however beneficial, met with some resistance because of the concern that psychiatric patients should not be allowed such "privileges." Another concern was that some of these patients had been productive workers throughout the hospital in assisting employees and had done so without remuneration. These concerns did not mar the positive responses to my work at the Togus VAMC, including the fact that I passed the psychiatry certification examination.

Frankly, my initial response to becoming a chief of staff trainee was to refuse because I preferred direct patient treatment rather than administration. Besides, I was happy working with our teams of dedicated workers. Yet I was intrigued by the challenge of having greater opportunities to help make a difference in the treatment and rehabilitation of more psychiatric patients. In such a dilemma, a change always involves difficult choices. When the chief of psychiatry service prepared to return to the central office, he asked me to call him as soon as possible so that arrangements could be initiated for my training.

In the end, my wife, an influential person for me, said that she would be willing to abide by whatever decision I made. She said that she believed

God would reveal to me what was best. With much ambivalence, I accepted the offer and was transferred to the VAMC in Lyons, New Jersey, in July 1961 for a year of job-apprentice training. Near the end of the training period, I was notified that I would be assigned to the VAMC in Tuskegee, Alabama.

Tuskegee

I knew the VAMC in Tuskegee was a unique facility. It was the only medical center in the VA system of 172 hospitals that was constructed exclusively for black veterans. Tuskegee VAMC opened on February 12, 1923, largely as a neuropsychiatric facility. This hospital was established and operated along racial lines. For many years it was the only VA medical facility where blacks could hold top management positions. Although health care for veterans is one of the major concerns of the Veterans Administration (now known as the Department of Veterans Affairs), it is ever sensitive and responsive to the political and social climate of the nation. Blacks have participated in all wars in which this county has been engaged. Yet the treatment and care of black veterans prior to the opening of Tuskegee VAMC was regarded as unorganized, even primitive, especially in the South, where the majority of black World War II veterans resided. The U.S. Congress proposed and authorized the location of a veterans hospital in the South. Repeated attempts to locate a community receptive to such a facility proved extremely difficult. In the absence of being allowed admission to certain veterans hospitals, especially for acute treatment, veterans were sent to military hospitals, often far from their homes, to obtain proper treatment. A narrative outlining some of the details of the development of the Tuskegee VAMC is found in Chapter 1 of this volume.

The 1950s and 1960s

During the late 1950s and into the 1960s, a tremendous turbulence (sometimes called a revolution) arose in U.S. social, political, economic, and cultural arenas. Radical changes in policies and practices of discrimination and segregation were being demanded. The American dream with regard to blacks could no longer be deferred. In 1962, Howard Kenney, M.D., an internist, made national news when he was appointed the first black hospital director outside Tuskegee VAMC. He was assigned to the VAMC in East Orange, New Jersey. Shortly after the Kenney appointment, I was selected to become the first black chief of staff at the VAMC in Northampton, Massachusetts, rather than at Tuskegee, as had been planned previously. I began this assignment in July 1962.

While at Northampton VAMC, I undertook strenuous efforts to recruit physicians, especially psychiatrists. Those already on staff were encouraged to engage in training programs to update their skills and to join the local medical society. Our hospital participated in a series of two-way telebroadcasts of medical programs that were transmitted from the Boston area to remote facilities. Generally, these meetings were well attended and included physicians from the community. I was one of the charter psychiatrists who helped to organize the Western Massachusetts Society (Chapter) of the New England branch of the American Psychiatric Association.

While attending my first VA regional meeting as "the new kid on the block," the regional director of psychiatry introduced me and asked me to give a report on the program at the Northampton VAMC. Being naive, I proudly mentioned that we had instituted a 20-bed treatment unit for psychiatric patients who also had addiction to alcohol, other drugs, or both. This report was not well received. I was told, in no uncertain terms, that not only was I violating VA policies, but to have the nerve to admit it at this meeting was beyond comprehension! After the meeting, several colleagues told me that they were also treating alcoholics and other drug addicts but would never mention this publicly. To do so could spell doom for one's future. I received the support of the hospital director, a psychiatrist, and did not abolish the program. Not long after this incident, the central office began to recommend establishing alcohol and drug treatment units in the local VA medical centers.

As a result of my hiring two well-qualified doctors of osteopathy, a consultant threatened to have me barred from the local medical society. Even though VA policies permitted the hiring of doctors of osteopathy, this consultant was opposed to this practice under any circumstances. The physicians remained on the staff, and I was not barred from the local medical society.

I was appointed a clinical assistant professor of psychiatry at the Albany Medical School. Two residents with whom I had worked joined the VA upon completion of their training. During my stay at Northampton VAMC, I had many opportunities to participate in several health-related groups and to speak or serve with various civic and religious organizations. I assisted in teaching registered nurses who were seeking master's degrees in nursing at the University of Massachusetts.

While at Northampton, one of the most surprising experiences that I, a Baptist, had was to be accused, along with the hospital director, who was Jewish, and the assistant director, an Irish Catholic, of discrimination against blacks in our hiring practices. This charge came from an Equal Employment Opportunity (EEO) investigator, who had found very few black employees at the medical center. The investigator was shown a record of our recruitment efforts and advised that there were only two blacks in the city of Northampton other than those who were either faculty or students at Smith College. Housing for blacks in Northampton was extremely limited. Several black families resided in the city of Holyoke, only 6 miles away. These residents were employed largely in nonprofessional, nonunionized jobs. Surveys indicated that their salaries were significantly higher than those we were paying for unskilled workers. In the past, nonmonetary appeals had little effect in attracting these workers to the hospital. Nevertheless, renewed efforts resulted in the hiring of two additional black employees. The EEO investigator was satisfied with our renewed efforts.

Battle Creek

In August 1967 I was notified that the administrator of the VA wanted to appoint me hospital director of the VAMC in Battle Creek, Michigan. At that time, the current director was in the process of retiring and had already moved out of the house on the hospital grounds. Initially, I was to assume the awesome and dual capacities od acting hospital director and chief of staff. I began this assignment with a deep sense of humility and commitment in September 1967.

Rumors exist in most organizations. This was certainly the case when I went to Battle Creek. There was widespread fear among employees that I had been sent to this facility to close it. Why else would the central office send a black man there? No blacks had ever been in any top management positions before. One day a group of black employees came to see me to request some favors. They announced, "You obviously have a lot of political pull; otherwise, you would never be here." As I attempted to direct the discussion to their concerns and the alleged "political pull" they thought I had, the employees said they had seen pictures of the new VAMC to be built in Detroit. Because many of our patients were from Detroit, the employees had concluded that there would be no need for the hospital in Battle Creek. They wanted me to help arrange for them to get jobs at the Detroit facility.

The group became irritated with me when I attempted to reassure them that the VAMC in Battle Creek was not closing and that I did not have the "political pull" they thought I had. No words could persuade them. As they left, they again declared that no black would be sent to Battle Creek if the hospital was to remain open, but they would "get along" if I did not want to help them. Working to overcome the low morale and hostility that I experienced during the initial phase of my stay in Battle Creek required tremendous efforts. Greetings were often polite but rather cool.

The decor of the office of the hospital director did little to brighten my reception to the facility. The walls of this large room had been papered with a dark brown material, simulating wood paneling. A huge desk and chair were placed on one side of the room, and a long, wide table with several chairs was on the other side. There were no attractive pictures on the wall, and the drapes on the windows had witnessed many sunrises and sunsets. An old coatrack that could accommodate about four coats stood by the door. The adjoining secretary's office was large enough to contain an old metal desk, two chairs, and two file cabinets. The office of the chief of staff also had an old metal desk (on which there were several old papers and manuals) and a chair with a missing roller. The knob for the radiator was missing, and a throw rug covered a hole in the middle of the floor. A rotten apple was clearly visible in the bookcase behind the desk. A torn shade hung at the single window.

There were approximately 1,300 patients in the hospital; many of them were indeed from the Detroit area—140 miles away. They passed two other VAMCs, which were designated as acute hospitals, en route to Battle Creek. The patients at our hospital were thought to require long-term psychiatric care. A good portion of them were in need of treatment for alcohol and other drug addiction (the same old problem that had long existed throughout the VA). On staff were 12 physicians, two of whom had had training in psychiatry. Approximately 63 registered nurses were among the total of 1,000 employees to provide the treatment. The one consultant in psychiatry made a monthly visit to the hospital and saw two or three patients per visit.

Shortly after my arrival in Battle Creek, I was assigned to gather sufficient data to help the central office determine the needs by 1980 for neuropsychiatric beds in the lower peninsula of Michigan. The report was to be into the central office within 4 months! At first I thought this was a joke, but I soon learned that it was not. The report was submitted on time.

The accrediting agency for hospitals, the Joint Commission for Accreditation of Health Organizations (JCAHO), was scheduled for a visit within 6 months of my appointment. The head of the JCAHO team visited my office upon his arrival. While there, he flipped a coin, which struck the acoustical tile in the ceiling. He said, "Doctor, see that dent the coin made in that tile? I do not care how good your treatment of patients is—if that asbestos tile exists in any patient-care areas, there is no way you can pass this inspection." Needless to say, that same type of asbestos acoustical tile existed throughout the hospital. Several requests for funds to remove the tile were documented prior to my assignment at the hospital. These requests had not been approved. At that time, if a VA facility failed a JCAHO accreditation survey, the evaluation was considered unfavorable. I asked the JCAHO team leader to make reference in his report to the existence of the asbestos tiles as a significant reason for our failure to pass the evaluation. He did so. We were placed on probation for failing the accreditation survey. We received the necessary funds from the central office to remove the tile. Upon the revisit by the JCAHO team two years later, we received full accreditation with compliments (commendations for significant improvements). Additional funding also enabled us to improve our staffing, update equipment, institute improved treatment programs, and improve the general appearance of patient areas. Much of the overcrowding was relieved.

Shortly after the first visit by the JCAHO, I requested a trip to the central office to meet with the VA administrator, chief medical director, and certain department heads to discuss my more than 45 "number-one" priorities. Several of these requests were granted almost immediately, with the promise that the others would receive immediate "careful consideration."

I made weekly rounds about the hospital and grounds, including shops, laundry, and various clinics. Staff were notified ahead of time about these rounds; other rounds were impromptu. I usually had key personnel with me on the scheduled rounds. This facilitated decision making on-site. My visits would take place at various hours, on weekends, and on each shift. I became known as "the walking chief." My willingness to meet regularly with the president of the employees' union, conduct regular staff meetings, and deal forthrightly with staff members' concerns brought about a shift in their attitudes, from the initial negative reactions to positive support.

In addition to meeting with employees, I arranged to meet with my counterparts at the VAMCs in nearby communities—Ann Arbor, Allen Park, Saginaw, and the outpatient clinic in Detroit. Also, I arranged to meet with the mayor; the director of the local hospitals; the police chief and the fire chief; the superintendent of schools; local school principals; judges; individuals from the news media; civic, business, and religious leaders; representatives of various service and volunteer groups; the president of the Chamber of Commerce; my counterpart at the Federal Civil Defense Unit; and the commander at nearby Fort Custer Military Base. These public relations endeavors helped tremendously in gaining considerable understanding and support for our treatment and rehabilitation programs, such as having patients who were significantly recovered living in selected homes in the community. Various businesses began to hire patients. We were able to arrange for buses to extend their services to transport patients as well as relatives, visitors, and employees to and from the city and the hospital. The news media published more balanced accounts of activities involving the hospital or patients. One account referred to a "quiet revolution" taking place at the hospital. The 600 volunteers and veterans service organizations were extremely dedicated to assisting in the treatment, recreation, and rehabilitation efforts. The administrator of the VA made two visits to VAMC at Battle Creek. According to the employees, this was a first-time occurrence.

During the time I was in Battle Creek, there was the widely expressed commitment throughout the Department of Veterans Affairs to make "the treatment of veterans second to none." It was a real sense of pride to be identified with that spirit.

With additional support in funding we were able to increase staff; however, we did not reach the magical ratio of one employee to one patient. Additional psychiatric consultants and visits enabled us to do much-needed in-service training. Supplemental training support came from pharmaceutical companies, a practice that was permitted at that time. The removal of high barbed-wire fences and bars from windows of most buildings and the use of bright colors, new equipment, and new furnishings in the living areas helped to enhance a therapeutic environment. A proposal that was directed to the central office outlined a plan for centralization in Battle Creek of all laundry facilities in the Lower Peninsula. The proposal, which was viewed to save costs, was accepted.

We opened a 167-bed unit for the treatment of alcohol and other drug addiction. This was one of the largest such units in the VA system. As was anticipated, there were outcries from within and outside the hospital that having such a unit would distract from the treatment of "real" psychiatric patients and attract a "bunch of addicts." The chief psychologist and a physician-consultant were placed in charge of the facility. The staff took a training course with recurrent updates. Throughout the hospital, patients' lengths of stay began to be markedly reduced.

We were able to arrange for medical students from the University of Michigan to come to the hospital with their instructors and participate in the patient training programs. I was appointed clinical professor in psychiatry at Michigan State University. Several nursing assistants were selected to train (with full financing) at a local college to become registered nurses. Through our efforts, an outstanding physician, who happened to be an osteopathic doctor, was accepted for a 3-month orientation in psychiatry at

VAMC in Topeka. His performance made such an impression that he was accepted for a full 3-year residency training program in psychiatry. Later he was appointed to a chief of staff position, the first osteopathic physician to hold that position at a VA hospital.

I was appointed to chair a committee to recruit blacks for middle- and top-management positions. We achievd some modest degree of success. One of those recruited, Viola Johnson, who first trained as a dietitian, became one of the few female hospital directors. Another of the recruits, David Whatley, progressively advanced and is currently a regional director responsible for approximately 24 VAMCs.

On the day that Martin Luther King Jr. was assassinated, there was a great uproar at the hospital with strong racial overtones. Some employees immediately lowered the U.S. flag to half-mast. No one seemed concerned about work. I asked the chaplains to conduct a "healing service" in the chapel. All employees were invited, and the chapel overflowed. Much of the tension was defused amid tears and expressions of deep sorrow, anger, and hurt.

It has been 22 years since I left the VAMC in Battle Creek. Yet the rumors persist that this facility is slated for closing. (Indeed, the much-talked-about VAMC in downtown Detroit is currently under construction.) It was my privilege to serve on the state and local committees for Hire the Handicapped; the United Way; and various school, religious, and civic committees. The highest award the city of Battle Creek bestows upon a citizen for voluntary service is known as the George Award (as in "Let George do it"). It came as a great surprise, but a real honor, to be the recipient of this award a few days before I departed (in June, 1973) for my next assignment.

Brockton, Massachusetts

I began my assignment as hospital administrator in Brockton in July 1973. One of the distinctive features about the VA facility there was that it was designed to have a bed capacity not to exceed 1,000. Considering that psychiatric hospitals sometimes had bed capacities of 1,500 to 2,000, were not affiliated with any medical school, were located in isolated areas, and were understaffed and frequently underfunded, that was a highly desirable factor. The original director of that VAMC is the one I succeeded. Contrary to the practice of transferring many of the directors every 3 or 5 years, he had remained in his position for 16 years. Again, I was the first black to be appointed to the position of hospital director there.

A few days after my arrival, a news reporter from the local press came to follow up on a particular story about the hospital. When my secretary brought him into my office, I stood to introduce myself. He stopped just inside the office with a look of astonishment and said, "You are the hospital director?" In response to my affirmative reply, he commented, "But you're black. I wonder if the folks in town know about this. I have never heard of a VA director who is black." I confirmed his statement by saying, "I am black." I added that a front-page story in his own paper had carried a photograph of me upon my arrival. I suggested that he might wish to read the article. Also, I informed him that there were other directors of VA facilities who are black. I inquired if he wanted to discuss his original purpose for visiting the hospital or spend our time discussing his concerns about my presence as the director. He said he could check on the original purpose of his visit some other time. He wanted to write something about me. I told him that I was not desirous of any personal publicity. I added that I hoped the local paper had been printing balanced accounts of hospital-related matters. He persisted in seeking information about me and said that I had "some mighty big shoes to fill because your predecessor was highly regarded in the community." I informed the reporter that I had known my predecessor for several years and that I too held him in high regard. Pointing to my shoes, I said, "I walk in no one's shoes but my own." The caption of the his article read, "New Director at Brockton VAMC to Walk in His Own Shoes."

Overall, I was well received by staff, general employees, patients, volunteers, and the community. Many therapeutic programs were already in place. Although staffing was only fair, it was a vast improvement over the pattern that had existed at other facilities where I had served.

Perhaps the most immediate task facing me initially was to pursue all factors pertaining to the opening of a 100-bed spinal cord rehabilitative unit on schedule. The resident engineer brought multiple construction flaws to my attention. I notified an unhappy central office of these defects and recommended that they be corrected and the scheduled opening delayed. The central office sent a team of eight engineers to look into the matter. After the complaint had been verified, the date of the opening was rescheduled. After the ceremonies were concluded I asked the engineer (who had headed the inspection team), in a private exchange, what would have happened if the defects had not been corrected. He responded, "There would have been hell to pay." As had been done at the VAMC in Battle Creek, the proposal to consolidate certain laundries in the district was accepted. Thus thousands of dollars were saved.

An externship program involving medical students from Harvard, Boston University, and Tufts was developed, utilizing board-certified staff and consultant psychiatrists. We developed a fairly comprehensive syllabus for this program. Some students received credit for the 2-month psychiatry rotation. I served on the dean's committee of Harvard University Medical School, with whom VAMC of Brockton was affiliated.

As part of the endeavor to promote more-positive relations between the people of the community and the patients at the hospital, we developed a grandparent-child program. Working with the superintendent of schools, teachers, parents, and the principal of a local school, we started this program with fourth- and fifth-graders coming to the hospital twice weekly to meet with senior-age patients. The teachers and staff worked closely with the participants. Volunteers were outstanding in their assistance. A local civic organization provided bus transportation for the students. Geography, history, science, and recreational activities were included in the program. The patients looked forward to the days their "grands" were to visit the hospital.

A good deal of effort was necessary to overcome some of the difficulties that existed in obtaining contracts, even the set asides, for minorities in business. Some significant progress became apparent after several months of diligent undertaking. Many "notables" in various fields, especially sports, politics, and the military, accepted invitations to visit the veterans. It was my good fortune to work closely with the other VAMC directors in the New England area while at the Brockton VAMC. I was appointed by the central office to serve on various special task forces. These assignments often involved a good deal of travel. For quite a while, the VA had been experiencing major losses of psychiatric registered nurses and nursing assistants. Some of these positions were difficult to fill. Despite arguments to the contrary, many of these employees were attracted to jobs outside the VA system that paid better salaries and had comparable benefits. I was selected by the chief medical director in the central office to come to Washington (along with eight other physician directors and one nonmedical hospital director) to testify before the House Veterans Affairs Committee. The testimonies pertained to a bill that would raise salaries of essential categories of employees in an attempt to retain employees and improve recruitment. About 2 weeks later I was asked to return to Washington to testify for this bill before the Veterans Committee of the U.S. Senate.

Although the bill passed, it excluded physicians who were hospital directors. These physicians were offered the choice of accepting a downgrade to a position of chief of staff, chief of psychiatry, or perhaps a ward physician. This downgrading would allow us to be eligible for the raise. Of course, we were free to remain as we were.

When physician board certification was deleted as a requirement for directorship of a psychiatric facility, an expanded and new breed of staff arose:

nonphysician hospital administrators. Another factor in their rise to prominence was that many physicians were reluctant to become administrators. The "old guard" was mostly displaced. The majority of physician directors stepped down. I was offered a position as associate chief in the Department of Psychiatry in VACO in Washington. Once again, I encountered ambivalence in changing to a position that removed me further from direct patient care. However, after much deliberation I accepted the offer and left Brockton in March 1976.

VA Central Office

> Let us . . . care for him who shall have borne the battle and for his widow and his orphan.

These words, from President Lincoln's second inaugural address, are engraved on a plaque affixed to the front of the building of the central office and set the basis for the mission of the VA.

In my new position, I participated in developing, coordinating, reviewing, and evaluating treatment modalities and programs for psychiatric patients and veterans addicted to alcohol, other drugs, or both nationwide. To go from concerns pertaining to a local VAMC to a systemwide setting presented another significant adjustment. Certainly all of one's previous experiences are brought to bear in this role. Duties covered a variety of general as well as specific assignments with much paperwork management and countless committee meetings. I reviewed volumes upon volumes of clinical folders in order to recommend a response to veterans' requests for changes in either their diagnosis or their service-connected disability. I participated indrafting and updating policies and manuals pertaining to psychiatric treatment; sharing in the interviewing of candidates for top management positions (e.g., chief of psychiatry, heads of departments in the central office); assisting with the search for answers to particular matters at local VAMCs; and preparing letters in response to inquiries from politicians at various levels, veterans, business or professional organizations, and individual citizens. One of my specific assignments dealt with maintaining statistics and preparing reports on assaults and suicides throughout the system. For several years I served as the VA representative to the National Institute of Mental Health's Committee on Mental Health. Frequent assignments of my job in the central office included investigation of a specific problem or determination of a facility's readiness for a JCAHO evaluation. I carried out these investigations as a member of a team or individually. As so often is the case in a large bureaucratic organization, frequently I never knew if the recommendations were actually implemented.

I had several opportunities to work with other departments within the central office, including nursing, chaplains, podiatry, pathology, social service, Equal Employment Opportunity, and voluntary services. The Department of Psychiatry encouraged continuing education activities and indeed helped to fund attendance at some meetings of national associations. For 4 years, I served as a clinical assistant professor of psychiatry at Howard University Medical School. I also served as a mentor with some of the inner-city youth at Eastern High School. In addition, I served on the original committee to institute programs related to black history observances in the central office.

In the early 1980s there was a period of much unrest as the veterans of the Vietnam War became irritated and distrustful of the "power structure in Washington." It became necessary to post guards at the entrance to the central office; passes or identification badges were required for entry. The veterans were demanding better recognition for their efforts in Vietnam, better benefits, rehabilitation, and treatment programs, including for alcohol and drug addiction. These demands were especially related to being diagnosed as having posttraumatic stress disorder and their desire for nonmedical and outpatient treatment for alcohol and other drug addictions.

Cries for funds for new programs, research, or the continuation of successful programs could be heard throughout the VA. The opportunity to sit in on the deliberations of various congressional committees provided some enlightenment as to why certain actions were being taken. This, however, did not lessen the impact of the reduction in funds and the consequent services to veterans.

Upon Retiring

Throughout my career, support provided by staff in the workplace and my family paved the way for a number of successes. My style of administration, which promoted upward mobility among the staff, served to foster good rapport as well as to further the efficiency of operation of the facility and assure that patients received sound and effective health care services. "Family pow-wows," which preceded each move, served to lessen the disquiet that our children sometimes experienced and fostered some excitement and pleasure about the move to a new locale. Certainly my wife was the prime contributor to the smoothness of the moves as experienced by the family.

The problems (e.g., expressions and patterns of racial discrimination, staff and community resistance to change) that I encountered in the workplace were irritants but did not distract me from planning and instituting changes that I thought would be in the best interest of the patients. I am pleased to have effected a number of changes. Among them, I am most proud to have created a therapeutic environment (i.e., ordering the removal of bars from the windows in some facilities; moving from a custodial to a treatment environment), establishing alcohol and drug-treatment programs, and developing good relations with the local media and the community in which we lived and worked. Also it was my privilege to help provide upward mobility for several employees.

The course of my employment as a career psychiatrist in the Veterans Administration was completed after 33 years. I retired on January 31, 1986. The Distinguished Service Award was presented to me on behalf of the administrator of Veterans Affairs at that time. Receiving this honor was a memorable way of ending my federal service.

Editor's Note

At the beginning of this project, the editor contacted Dr. Baker to invite him to write a chapter on the experiences of black psychiatrists who chose the VA system as their career path. He accepted with only minimal hesitation, and together, we began the pursuit of data collection. It had been our initial plan to write to all black psychiatrists in the VA system and ask each one for information about their respective experiences. In short order, we learned that such a list did not exist, or at least was not available to us. Many, if not most, of our colleagues who were affiliated with the VA were informed of the project and invited to contact the editor if they wished to participate. Only a very few followed up on the matter, and we continued to fret about the sparsity of data.

We made direct contact with colleagues whom we knew to be associated with the VA, but the few responses we received did not diminish our concerns about the limited data that was available to the author. This called for several additional telephone conferences, which led to a modification of the original plan; that is, the author would write from an autobiographical frame of reference. Dr. Baker, who has been and continues to serve as a role model for many of our younger colleagues, has provided an interesting and absorbing account of his experiences in the VA system. Readers who have selected the VA system as their career path are likely to find that some of Baker's experiences parallel their own.

PART IV

Current Mental Health Issues Affecting Black Americans

CHAPTER **14**

Current Mental Health Issues Affecting Black Americans

BILLY E. JONES, M.D., M.S.

The current mental health issues affecting black Americans are many. Most affect both provider and consumer, psychiatrist and patient. Some are new, but most, like institutionalized racism, are continuing problems that have never been resolved. Many of these issues are not germane to mental health care alone; rather they are generic to all American health care, medical education, and research. Mental health issues all too often reflect broader concerns in American society and culture and mirror the accomplishments and failures of our society (Griffith 1986). The field of mental health is no better, and probably no worse.

This chapter will discuss contemporary issues affecting black Americans. It begins with a brief overview of health care reform and then discusses how reform will affect both black American psychiatrists and psychiatric patients. Some of the issues raised in the chapter are new. They are the direct consequences of reform. Others have existed for many years but will be deeply affected by the transformation of American health care.

Health Care Reform

Today, Americans confront a rapidly and radically changing health care environment that is affecting providers and consumers alike. Mental health care is changing quickly. How services are provided, how care is financed, who provides that care, and who will get it are being discussed, debated, and implemented. What is clear is that health care reform is the lens through which nearly every contemporary issue in all of medicine must be viewed.

These changes are having a profound impact on black American psychiatrists and patients. In some instances the consequences of health care reform are similar to those affecting white Americans; in other instances they are quite different. Change always creates misgivings, doubts, and fears, and clearly the forces transforming health care are producing a good deal of anxiety.

Black American providers worry about their future as professionals. Heretofore, black physicians have earned respectable salaries, though not always the equivalent of their white counterparts. Doctors have been at the upper levels of the black American socioeconomic ladder. It has been economically desirable for a black person to aspire to be a doctor. Both earnings and security have been nearly assured. Now, in the midst of change, black American physicians worry if they will have a job. Those in training worry if they will find positions in the future. All worry about the continuing earning capacity of black doctors. As a result, many black doctors are advising their children to seek other careers.

In years past, most black American psychiatrists had the option of creating a private practice in minority communities or working in a public mental health agency. Many did both. With health care reform, financing for private psychiatric practice is drying up and public mental health agencies are downsizing or being phased out. With fewer jobs for psychiatrists, black American psychiatrists have more to worry about than their white counterparts. The last hired, first fired adage, though not applicable to black American psychiatrists in the past, now seems to be increasingly pertinent to our lives.

Black American consumers, or patients, are likewise affected by the changing health care environment. Controls on the health care dollar raise fears about the availability of needed care. Mental health services for black Americans have never been adequate or readily assessable. The present dollar-driven reforms both fail to address this situation and threaten to aggravate it by restricting utilization and limiting who will receive treatment. Black American mental health care consumers with health care insurance will be limited because most insurances are restricting mental health coverage. Those on Medicaid and Medicare are worried as state after state as well as the federal government make drastic reductions and changes in these entitlement programs. Finally, black Americans without any coverage who have gotten care through a variety of funding mechanisms are watching states dismantle these arrangements for uncompensated care without creating viable alternative plans. Black consumers are concerned about a future that promises a lack of treatment, financial restrictions, and a lack of appropriate, culturally competent services.

Selecting Psychiatry as a Career/Selecting Mental Health Services

One of the most important current issues in psychiatry affecting black Americans is the reluctance of blacks to become involved with psychiatry. Too few black Americans practice psychiatry and too few seek treatment. Health care reform will not resolve this problem and could well exacerbate it.

Becoming a Psychiatrist

For black physicians, selecting psychiatry as a career is an unpopular choice. Though the reasons for this are not totally clear, some are intrinsic to the black experience whereas others are external. Status, earning power, perceived need, perceived use to the black American community, and lack of adequate role models are only a few of the reasons that black doctors do not become psychiatrists.

There is much in the black experience that deters young doctors from pursuing psychiatry. As in other communities, being a physician carries a certain degree of status. Doctors are seen as men and women of action. The image of a doctor is that of a healer who carries a black bag and acts to treat an illness. Although the doctor talks to and interacts with the patient, the aim is to *physically* heal a wound, cure a cold, or set a fracture. All are active, assertive acts. To treat an illness through verbal interactions is not a part of the conceptual structure of what a doctor is. It is seen as passive. Black physicians come to training with this conceptual structure. Unless efforts are made to change and expand this concept, black doctors in training continue not to consider psychiatry as a viable career choice.

The failure to enhance the status of psychiatrists in the black American community can be seen in the relationship of black colleagues in other specialties to black psychiatrists. Many black doctors hold psychiatry in less esteem than the other specialties and are not supportive of the field. They often fail to refer black American patients to psychiatrists and attempt to treat psychiatric illnesses themselves.

Efforts to include capable, interested black American psychiatrists as role models in medical school training programs have been too few and too halfhearted. It is highly likely that health care reform will provide few incentives to raise the status of black American psychiatrists. Managed care and the need to save dollars will, in all probability, work to increase biases in the black community against psychiatry.

Becoming a Patient

Much has been written about the mental health help-seeking behavior of black Americans (Neighbors 1988). It is the author's observation that over the past 10 to 15 years black Americans have become more cognizant of psychological issues and needs. The media, medical and other health care professions, music, religion, and black leaders have all played a part in this development. Though there is a greater sense of readiness to seek and accept treatment, it does not always become operationalized because of many external, environmental obstacles.

Environmental factors continue to serve as obstacles for black Americans in seeking mental health services. For some, the struggle to meet basic needs leaves little time to seek help for emotional and psychological problems. The struggle has not become easier. With welfare cutbacks and increased job losses in a decreased job market, the prospect of avoiding life on the edge for many black American would-be mental health consumers is not good. The lack of available community-based mental health resources makes accessibility a continuing issue for others. With government at all levels redefining and downsizing their roles, the publicly funded, community-based mental health treatment services will become less available and less accessible. A shortage of culturally competent services exists for all too many black Americans (Jones and Smith 1997). Although this problem has been recognized, a sustained effort at educating all providers to make them culturally competent is far from completion.

Managed Care

The reform of health care has arrived and it is named managed care. Insurances, businesses, and provider entities are making the decisions regarding financial reimbursement for health services rendered. These entities have entered into risk-sharing contracts with employers, governments, or both to manage the health care and costs of their employees or eligible covered lives. In some instances this is done through health maintenance organizations, from which the patient must receive all care. Other plans include panels of preselected physicians, networks of services that the patients use, or a combination of those plans. In these arrangements, the providers have agreed to use certain protocols and criteria for admission and for the type and length of treatment. Prospective and retrospective reviews and audits are an important part of this arrangement. Behavioral managed-care companies contract directly with employers and governments or subcontract with general health care entities to manage the behavioral care.

There are considerable pros and cons about managed care and some of the associated practices. However, reform is controlling costs and is here to stay. Managed care has become a current and new mental health issue affecting black Americans.

The Impact on Black Psychiatrists

Although some concerns about managed care may be general to all psychiatrists, black American psychiatrists have some specific issues. Many of these are shared with black physicians in general. Most arise from being a minority in this country, in medicine and in psychiatry. A large percentage of black American physicians feel that they are not included in the formation of health care policies and that they face high levels of professional and health care system racial discrimination (Byrd et al. 1994).

Black American psychiatrists have not been actively and equitably included in most of the previous movements and changes in psychiatry. Will they be included in panels and provider networks in managed care? Though the exclusion may come as a result of omission, not commission, black Americans will be left out if special consideration is not given to including minorities in these areas. Because there are few black psychiatrists, the regular mechanisms of selecting panels and networks are unlikely to reach and include them. Like other black physicians, most black psychiatrists have practiced in solo or small group arrangements, in inner cities or in rural, underserved communities. Managed care is in many ways contrary to this environment in that it encourages and works best with physicians operating in large groups (Walton 1995). In addition, solo practitioners have limited impact on the decision-making process of these organizations. Special outreach and recruitment by the managed care companies is necessary. These special efforts may not fit with the profit incentive to control and limit costs.

In addition to inclusion, there is the issue of involvement of black American psychiatrists at senior levels within the behavioral managed care companies. Few of the companies have black American psychiatrists in senior policy and decision-making positions. As Medicaid managed care further evolves and more black American patients join or are forced into these plans, the need for such policy makers increases. The need is not just to represent the population the company is serving, but also for the knowledge and skill base the black American psychiatrists will bring. They can speak to the needs of black American patients, in the areas of both culturally competent treatment and program planning.

The Impact on Black Patients

There is much concern about psychiatric patients in managed care. This has centered around the issue of which conditions are covered in the plan and which are not. Not much attention has been focused on the needs of different ethnic and racial groups for culturally competent treatment. Nor has there been a focus on how to incorporate such treatment into the menu of services made available. Black American patients will continue to need and should receive community-based, culturally competent care. Black American children and adolescents should receive care through a family-centered approach provided by school- and community-based treatment programs (Cross et al. 1989).

Though all black American mental health patients need culturally competent care, other needs may vary. Medicaid recipients need accessible and available services. Those with no mental health care coverage need services.

Academe/Research

For many years the gold standard of psychiatry has been research and training in academia. The leaders in the field of psychiatry have come from academic and research institutions. Almost all have been white males. Even with few black psychiatrists, there has been a disproportionately small number of blacks in academic or research psychiatry. Moreover, only approximately 3% of medical school faculties are ethnic minorities (Baker 1993). Institutional racism is a continuing and current mental health issue affecting black Americans.

Black Psychiatrists

Several factors are thought to be related to the very small number of black Americans in academic or research psychiatry. Many feel that involvement in the direct care and treatment aspects of psychiatry is a more direct and concrete way to assist the black community. Thus, they seem to be more interested in the practice and treatment aspects of psychiatry than in research and training.

Both the research and academic area function on a mentor/apprentice model. The mentor serves many functions. He or she serves as a role model, visibly indicating that the student, too, can accomplish and be successful. The mentor serves as a sponsor, team leader, facilitator, and guide. He or she teaches the student the skills and culture of the field, guides the student around pitfalls and mistakes, and furthers the career and goals of the student. Only a very few of the white male psychiatrists, who have dominated these fields, have provided the guidance and direction necessary to encourage and allow black psychiatrists to negotiate the steps leading to successful careers in academia, research, or both. With few black researchers and academicians, there have been a very limited number of black mentors available for young black psychiatrists as role models and sponsors. Admission to these fields has been nearly closed while guidance, support, and furtherance of the careers of interested young black psychiatrists have been rare.

Black Patients

Much has been written about the health status of black Americans and the continuing dilemma and flawed efforts to mainstream black Americans into the health system (Byrd and Clayton 1992). "At no time in history has the health of black Americans equalled that of white Americans" (Charatz-Litt 1992). This statement is equally true, though less known, about mental health. Yet this fact has failed to garner an interest or focus on mental health issues and black Americans by the psychiatric academic or research community. There has been a singularly striking lack of interest, whether in looking at ethnic and racial factors and difference in diagnosis, treatment response, and biological markers or the cultural determinants of illness (Carter 1994; Jones and Gray 1986; Lawson 1986). Although this is a continuing issue affecting black Americans, its significance at this time makes it a current issue as well. Today, those in academics and research in the general health arena recognize and acknowledge the health status differences and are making attempts to focus on corrective actions. In psychiatry, these differences are still generally ignored.

There is a lack of special focus on black American patients, even though they make up a considerable proportion of the public psychiatric patient population. A review of the psychiatric literature reveals a dearth of recent articles on black American patients or related issues. Those new contributions to the literature are mostly by black psychiatrists, with little done by others. Even when black patients are included in the research sample, they are rarely separated out for focus and discussion.

Most of the recent and older psychiatric literature about blacks has been done by black behavioral scientists. It is clear that the lack of a sufficient number of black psychiatrists in research and academic institutions and pursuits is directly related to little new focus and knowledge about black Americans and mental illness.

Organized Psychiatry

Issues affecting black Americans continue to be readily observable within organized psychiatry. Some of these issues are rooted in long-standing institutional racism. The history of black psychiatrists and the challenges to racism in organized psychiatry are well documented (Pierce 1973). As indicated in Chapter 1 of this volume, numerous and vigorous efforts have been directed toward the eradication of the inequities in professional organizations. Significant progress has been made, but some problems continue to exist.

Professional Organizations

Significant representation of black psychiatrists in the leadership ranks of professional organizations is yet to be accomplished. This is an important goal to be reached to insure true integration and input of the opinions and views of black Americans in the deliberations and policy making of the organizations. Often, issues of particular concern to black Americans do not get raised or addressed without the presence and voice of black representation. The role model and barrier-breaking effect is also vitally important, as it opens the door to full participation of additional black Americans and other minorities. Several psychiatric organizations will be mentioned to illustrate the continuing problem.

A black psychiatrist has never been elected to the office of president of the American Psychiatric Association, although two were candidates for the office (in 1976 and 1981). Three black psychiatrists were elected to the post of vice president (in 1980, 1973, and 1974), and one was twice (1976 and 1978) elected treasurer. Since the height of the civil rights era it appears to have been more difficult for a black American to win an election. Since 1980 no black psychiatrist has been named as a candidate for the office of president elect, vice president, secretary, or treasurer. The APA Assembly elected the first black and the first woman speaker-elect in 1997.

According to the APA membership office, there are currently (1998) 40,386 members of the association, 886 of whom are black Americans. Although black representation is a small percentage of the total membership, this did not appear to be a determining factor in the election process in the past. It is interesting to note that in other major medical associations with no greater percentage of black American representation (e.g., American Medical Association, American College of Physicians, American College of Surgeons, American Medical Women's Association) black physicians have been elected to the highest office.

Several black American neurologists have served as directors of the American Board of Psychiatry and Neurology (ABPN), but there has been only one black American psychiatrist who was elected to the board and one who was elected to the Committee on Certification in Child and Adolescent Psychiatry. Though the leadership area still needs concentrated attention, the ABPN has made considerable strides in increasing the number of black psychiatrists serving as examiners. Currently (1998), there is generally more than one per examining team. (The author has served as an examiner for the oral examinations for many years and over the last several years has not been the only black member on his team. Moreover, he was paired with another black American examiner in a 1996 examination).

Although the American College of Psychiatrists (ACP) is making efforts to recruit black psychiatrists into its membership, this is a recent event. The ACP, with an active membership of 600, has very few black American psychiatrists. None have been nominated or elected to a leadership position.

Affirmative Action

As the thinking and decision making of this country has moved to a decidedly more conservative position, support and implementation of affirmative action has weakened, waned, and almost vanished. In this overall climate blacks worry about the commitment of organized psychiatry to affirmative action. This represents another current issue affecting black Americans. Though all of the major professional organizations have affirmative action policies, will they continue to stress them with the pressure off? Much of the progress to date occurred during the Civil Rights era, and the zeal for a continued vigorous push has withered. Unfortunately, not enough change has occurred or become institutionalized in psychiatry to sustain lasting equal treatment and results. The playing field is still not level for black psychiatrists or patients. The commitment to affirmative action needs to be even stronger than before. It was easier to be committed when the rest of the country was. Organized psychiatry needs a stronger commitment now that much of the country has moved away from the principles of affirmative action.

Summary

This chapter has addressed some of the current mental health issues affecting black American psychiatrists and patients in today's health care reform environment. It has briefly examined institutional racism as it continues to exist in various areas of psychiatry. Areas that have improved and those still requiring attention have been noted. Psychiatry, in many ways a window, simply lets through all the views from our contemporary world.

References

Baker FM: The black academic psychiatrist [letter]. Acad Med 68:501, 1993

Byrd WM, Clayton LA: An American health dilemma: a history of blacks in the health system. J Natl Med Assoc 84:189–200, 1992

Byrd WM, Clayton LA, Kinchen K, et al: black-American physicians' views on health reform: results of a survey. J Natl Med Assoc 86:191–199, 1994

Carter J: Racism's impact on mental health. J Natl Med Assoc 86:543–547, 1994

Charatz-Litt C: A chronicle of racism: the effects of the white medical community on black health. J Natl Med Assoc 84:717–725, 1992

Cross TL, Bazron BJ, Dennis W, et al: Toward a Culturally Competent System of Care. A Monograph on Effective Services for Minority Children Who Are Severely Emotionally Disturbed. Child and Adolescent Service System Program (CASSP), 1989

Griffith EEH: Blacks and American psychiatry. Hosp Community Psychiatry 37(1):5, 1986

Jones BE, Smith AE: Mental health needs: underserved and increasing in complexity, in Removing Risk from Children. Edited by Carten A, Dumpson JR. Silver Spring, MD, Beckham House Publishers, 1997, pp 127–147

Jones BD, Gray BA: Problems in diagnosing schizophrenia and affective disorders among blacks. Hosp Community Psychiatry 37:61–65, 1986

Lawson WB: Racial and ethnic factors in psychiatric research. Hosp Community Psychiatry 37:50–53, 1986

Neighbors HW: The help-seeking behavior of black Americans. J Natl Med Assoc 80:1009–1012, 1988

Pierce C: The formation of the black psychiatrists of America, in Racism and Mental Health. Edited by Willie CV, Kramer BM, Brown, BS. Pittsburgh, PA, University of Pittsburgh Press, 1973, 525–554

Walton T: Challenges for health professionals in the face of health-care market reform. J Natl Med Assoc 87:256–257, 1995

Index

Abbott, Anderson, 96
Academia, and black psychiatrists. *See also* Education; Faculty; Medical schools; Meharry Medical College; Teaching
  gender differences in faculty positions, 125–26, 143
  medical school faculties and, 114–116, 118–120
  research and training in, 210–212
  survey of, 116–127
Adams, Milton, 130–131
Adams, Walter, 9
Administration, and black psychiatrists
  academia and, 121
  department of psychiatry at Harlem Hospital, 41–42
  Veterans Administration and, 200–201
Affective disorder, underdiagnosis of in blacks, 81
Affirmative action
  professional organizations in psychiatry and, 214
  public policy on mental health issues and, 60
Africa, observations of black psychiatrist from, on American psychiatry in 1970s and 1980s, 77, 91
Aftercare, and inpatient services in general hospital, 33
Albany Medical School, 192
Alcoholism treatment programs
  department of psychiatry at Harlem Hospital and, 42
  Harlem Rehabilitation Center and, 52
  New York State Office of Alcoholism Services, 62
  Veterans Administration and, 192, 196
Aldrich, C. Knight, 69
Alfred, Dewitt, 12, 13, 96–97

Alternative psychiatric care, and black patients, 85–86, 164
American Academy of Child and Adolescent Psychiatry, 21–22, 134, 138, 139
American Academy of Psychiatry and the Law, 158
American Academy of Psychoanalysis, 171, 172
American Board of Psychiatry and Neurology (ABPN), 20, 213
American College of Psychiatrists (ACP), 213
American Journal of Psychiatry, 4
American Orthopsychiatry Association (AOA), 21
American Psychiatric Association (APA)
  Assembly of District Branches, 17, 18, 138
  Black Caucus, 134
  Committee of Black Psychiatrists, 17–18, 20, 114
  forensic psychiatry and presentations at meetings of, 158
  history of black participation in, 4, 5–6, 8, 16–19
  leadership of and representation of black psychiatrists, 213
  number of black psychiatrists in membership of in 1995/1996, 173
  Offices of Minority/National Affairs and Research, 148
  Program for Minority Research Training in Psychiatry, 19, 148–149
  program for recruitment of minority students into psychiatry, 113–114
  Resident Census Data on black psychiatrists in 1989–1994, 115
  Western Massachusetts Society of New England branch of, 192

American Psychoanalytic Association, 137, 165, 171–172
American Public Health Association, 21
Anderson, John, 17
Anderson, Robert S., 67
Apartheid (South Africa), 17–18
Association of American Medical Colleges (AAMC), 110, 112–113
Assue, Claire, 13, 14
Augusta, Alexander, 96
Averbach, I. Jay, 37

Baker, James E., 187–202
Baldwin, Edward, 97
Ballard, Bruce L., 13, 14, 18, 37, 43, 114, 169
Balm in Gilead: Journey of a Healer (Lightfoot, 1988), 129–130
Barker, Prince, 5
Barton, Walter, 19
Batizy, Gunstav, 74
Battle Creek Veterans Administration Medical Center (Michigan), 193–197
Baylor University College of Medicine, 130
Bell, Carl, 18
Bell, Iverson, 13
Bell, James, 9, 21, 22, 129, 130
Bell Curve: Intelligence and Class Structure in American Life, The (Herrnstein & Murray, 1994), 89
Bellevue Hospital (New York), 26, 29
Benoit, Marilyn, 22
Berlin Army Hospital, 103
Bernard, Viola W., 40, 165
Biassey, E. L., 171
Bilingualism, and mental health policy in New York City, 61
Biographical sketches, of black psychiatrists
 Solomon Carter Fuller, 3–4
 Raphael Hernandez, 5–6
 Charles Prudhomme, 7–9
 Ernest Y. Williams, 6–7
Black Americans
 civil rights movement and studies of impact of racism on mental health of, 15
 current mental health issues affecting
  health care reform and, 205–207
  managed care and, 208–210
  psychiatric research and, 211–212
  psychiatry as a career and, 207–208
 early research on mental disorders in, 142, 212
 observations of black psychiatrist from Africa on mental health research in U.S. and, 80–87
 percentage of in prison population, 153
 recruitment of as medical students, 110–113
Black psychiatrists
 historical reviews
  biographical sketches of influential figures, 3–22
  community psychiatry and public policy on psychiatric services, 47–65
  development of department of psychiatry at Harlem Hospital, 25–44
  development of department of psychiatry at Meharry Medical College, 67–75
  military psychiatry and, 95–104
  observations of black psychiatrist from Africa on 1970s and 1980s, 77–91
 managed care and, 209–210
 personal reminiscences
  on career in Veterans Administration, 187–202
  of head of university department of psychiatry, 185–186
  of state commissioner of mental health, 179–85
 professional organizations and representation in leadership, 212–214
 representation of in academia and in research, 210–211
 status of in black community, 207
 surveys of
  academia and, 109–127
  child and adolescent psychiatrists and, 129–139

forensic psychiatry and, 153–159
psychoanalysis and, 163–174
research and, 141–149
Black Psychiatrists of America (BPA)
child psychiatry and, 134
civil rights movement and establishment of, 14–15, 20
history of black leadership of, 20–21
Black Rage (Cobbs & Grier, 1968), 15
Bland, Walter, 12
Bonner, Frances Jones, 14
Bonner, Jocelyn, 97
Booth, Martin, 131
Boston University School of Medicine, 4
Bowen, Clotilde Dent, 97, 100–101, 103
Bowers, Marion, 74
Bowie-Elder, Zelda, 9
Bradley, Omar, 8
Bradshaw, Walter, 12, 17–18, 169, 171
Bragg, Robert, 13
Branche, George, 4–5
Brock-Davies, Frances, 34
Brockton Veterans Administration Medical Center (Massachusetts), 197–200
Brown v. Board of Education of Topeka, Kansas (1954), 8, 48
Brown, George, 95
Bullock, Samuel C., 12, 169, 171
Butts, Hugh F., 15, 28, 31–32, 33, 42–43, 170, 171

Calhoun, Calvin, 14
Calhoun, Joshua W., 132, 133, 134, 135, 138
Campbell, Vivian, 97
Cannon, J. Alfred, 12, 13, 20
Carey, Hugh, 58
Carter, Jimmy, 64
Carter, Rosalyn, 64
Cassard, Lawrence, 28
Chandler, Delores, 34
Charles, Floyd, 97
Charles, Roderick, 14
Charles R. Drew Community Mental Health and Mental Retardation Center (Philadelphia), 84–85
Charles R. Drew Postgraduate Medical School (Los Angeles), 12–13, 118

Cheevers, Tonya, 97
Chester M. Pierce, M.D., Sc.D. Resident and Medical Student Research Symposium, 16
Child and adolescent psychiatry, and black psychiatrists
diagnostic and treatment patterns in, 135–136
education and training of, 131–134
future opportunities in, 138–139
influential figures in, 129–131
practice patterns and professional affiliations of, 136–138
racist practices and, 134–135
Children's Hospital (Denver), 137
Children's Television Workshop, 131
Christmas, June Jackson, 11, 13, 17, 21, 30, 34, 35, 36, 171
Civil Rights Act (1875), 3
Civil rights movement
black psychiatrists in academia and, 109–110
black psychiatrists and activism, 14–15, 20
community psychiatry and, 48
Harlem Rehabilitation Center and, 52
personal reminiscences on, 191–192
Civil War, and black Americans in military medical service, 95–96
Clifton T. Perkins Hospital (Maryland), 10–11
Clinical practice, and forensic psychiatry, 155. *See also* Practice
Cobbs, Price, 15
Coleman, Claude, 97
Colleges. *See* Academia; Education; specific institutions
Collins, James L., 12, 96, 98, 101–102, 103
Columbia University, 26–27, 40
Combat stress behaviors, and military psychiatry, 99–103
Comer, James, 14, 19, 20, 21, 111, 130
Commissioner of mental health, personal reminiscences of career as, 179–185
Community Mental Health Act (1963), 41
Community mental health centers, and geographical system, 181–182

Community psychiatry
 department of psychiatry of Harlem Hospital and, 40–41
 fiscal crisis in New York City and, 62–63
 Harlem Rehabilitation Center and, 49–65
 progress and problems of in 1970s, 64–65
 public policy and, 59–62
 service system for New York City, 57–59
 social change movement in 1960s and, 48–49
Conference on Psychoanalytic Education and Research, 172
Confidentiality, and military psychiatry, 98–99
Cooper, Joan, 13
Coopwood, William, 12
Coping skills, and psychosocial stresses experienced by blacks, 84
Countertransference, and black students of psychoanalysis, 167–168
Courts, and forensic psychiatry, 155
Critical events debriefings, and military psychiatry, 102
Crownsville State Hospital (Maryland), 10–11
Culture. *See also* Ethnicity
 child psychiatry and, 132
 community psychiatry and public policy, 60–62
 education of black psychiatrists and, 114
 judicial and correctional systems and insensitivity to issues of, 158
 observations of black psychiatrist from Africa on U.S. in 1970s and 1980s, 79–87
 psychiatric curricula and, 72
 psychoanalysis and, 168
Curtis, James L., 13, 14, 111

Davis, Amos, 12
Davis, Elizabeth B., 13, 28, 29–30, 47, 165, 169
Davis, Ramona, 20
Davis, William S., Jr., 130
Day hospital, and department of psychiatry at Harlem Hospital, 31–34
DeGrass, John Van Surly, 95–96
Delaney, Martin, 96
Delgado, Andrea, 18, 20, 21
Dementia, and hallucinations in blacks, 82
Demography
 of black psychiatrists in academia, 118–120
 future trends in U.S., 139
 women and minorities in psychiatry and, 147–148
Department of Health, Education and Welfare, 64
Departments of psychiatry, development of at Harlem Hospital
 administration and, 41–42
 community psychiatry and, 40–41
 consolidation of services, 42–44
 day hospital and inpatient services, 31–34
 early planning process for, 28–29
 establishment of, 25–27
 Harlem Rehabilitation Center and, 53
 interdepartmental relationships and, 38–39
 mission of, 27
 outpatient services and, 29–31
 rehabilitation services and, 34–35
 review procedures and, 39
 social services and, 35
 training of psychiatrists and allied professionals, 36–38
Depression, research on diagnosis of in blacks, 80–81
Desegregation. *See* Racism
Diagnosis
 child and adolescent psychiatry and, 135–136
 research on psychiatric disorders in blacks and, 80–83, 85
Dillan, Vince, 97
Distinguished Service Award (American Psychiatric Association), 19

Distinguished Service Award (Veterans Administration), 202
Domestic Peace Corps, 41
Douglas, Florence, 12
Drake, Carl, Jr., 20
Dudley, Richard, 18
Dumas, Michael O., 4
Durant, Nancy, 131

Education, medical and psychiatric. See also Academia; Faculty; Medical schools; Meharry Medical College; Teaching
  in child and adolescent psychiatry, 131–134
  department of psychiatry at Harlem Hospital, 36–38
  department of psychiatry at Meharry Medical College, 71–73
  in forensic psychiatry, 154
  historical review of, 12–14
  of mental health workers at Harlem Rehabilitation Center, 53–55
  in psychoanalysis, 164, 166–168
  Veterans Administration system and, 187–191
Educational Commission for Foreign Medical Graduates (ECFMG), 25
Edward, Henry, 96, 170
Edwards, Pauline, 32
Edwards, Roy, 186
Egri, Gladys, 35
Elam, Lloyd C., 12, 21, 69–75
Ellis, Harold, 26
Ellis, William, 96
Emory College of Medicine, 13
Epidemiologic Catchment Area study, and ethnic differences in community prevalence of mental disorders, 87
Equal Employment Opportunity (EEO), and Veterans Administration, 193
Erskine, Kenneth, 38
Erwin, Herbert, 16
Ethnicity. See also Culture
  anthropological use of term "race," 84
  diversity in child psychiatry and, 132
  health care policy and, 91

E. Y. Williams, M.D. Clinical Scholars of Distinction Award, 16

Faculty. See also Teaching
  medical schools and positions held by black psychiatrists, 114–116, 118–120
  of Meharry Medical College department of psychiatry, 73–74
  percentage of medical school positions held by minorities, 141, 211
Family, and black psychiatry, 163–164
Ferguson, Yvonne, 13, 18
Fields, Richard A., 6, 7, 20
Ford, Edna, 38
Forensic psychiatry, and black psychiatrists
  definition of, 153
  degrees of experience in, 154–155
  future of, 159
  teaching and, 158
  training and, 154
  work environments of, 155–158
Forte, William, 97
Foster Grandparent Program, 181
Freedman, Daniel, 17
Freedmen's Hospital (Washington, D. C.), 7, 10
Fuller, Lillian, 97
Fuller, Ruth L., 131–132, 134, 136–137, 165, 169
Fuller, Solomon Carter, 3–4, 141
Funding, of black research psychiatrists, 144–145, 146

Garmiza, Carol, 38
Gaston, John, 13, 18
General hospital, development of department of psychiatry
  administration and, 41–42
  community psychiatry and, 40–41
  consolidation of services, 42–44
  day hospital and inpatient services, 31–34
  early planning process for, 28–29
  establishment of, 25–27
  interdepartmental relationships and, 38–39

General hospital, development of department of psychiatry (*continued*)
  mission of, 27
  outpatient services and, 29–31
  rehabilitation services and, 34–35
  review procedures and, 39
  social services and, 35
  training of psychiatrists and allied professionals, 36–38
Genetics, and hypothesis for racial differences in violence, 90–91
Geographical system, for organization of community mental health care, 181–182
Gers, Seymour, 43
Gibson, Robert, 17
Giles, Roscoe C., 111
Givens, Regie, 97
Goldin, Victor, 36
Goodin, Kathleen, 28
Gore, Tony, 11
Grandparent-child program, 199
Green, Robert E., 95
Grier, William, 12, 15
Griffith, Charles, 7–8
Griffith, Ezra E. H., 20
Group for the Advancement of Psychiatry (GAP), 21
Group therapy program, at Harlem Hospital, 34, 41
Gullattee, Alyce, 15
Guyden, Thomas, 96

Haitian refugees, and mental health care, 18
Hallucinations, and schizophrenia in blacks, 82
Hamilton, John M., 11, 19
Harding, Warren G., 4
Harlem Child Study Center, 41
Harlem Hospital (New York)
  development of department of psychiatry, 25–44
  Harlem Rehabilitation Center and, 53
  Veterans Administration and psychiatric education, 188

Harlem Rehabilitation Center
  development of, 49–50
  New York City policies on mental health careers and services, 59
  philosophy of sociopsychiatric rehabilitation and, 50–51
  problems and progress of in first decade, 55–56
  program services of, 51–53
  training of mental health workers, 53–55
Harris, Hiawatha, 12, 20
Harris, Thelissa, 20
Harrison-Ross, Phyllis, 15, 20–21, 131
Harvard University Medical School, 111, 199
Hawley, Paul, 8
Hayes, Frank W., 13, 97, 98
Heacock, Don, 131
Health care. *See also* Mental health
  child psychiatric services and reform of, 139
  managed care and mental health services for black Americans, 208–210
  mental health services for black Americans and reform of, 205–207
  needs of black community and, 173
  psychiatric research and reform of, 148
  public policy and diversity in, 91
Henry, E. Pentoka, 9
Hernandez, Raphael, 5–6, 73, 74
Hines, Ralph, 74
History, of black psychiatrists and American psychiatry
  academia and, 109–116
  administrative and clinical psychiatrists and, 9–12
  biographical sketches of influential figures, 3–9
  civil rights movement and, 14–15
  development of department of psychiatry at Harlem Hospital, 25–44
  development of department of psychiatry at Meharry Medical College, 67–75

medical education and, 12–14
military psychiatry and, 95–104
observations of black psychiatrist from Africa on U.S. in 1970s and 1980s, 77–91
professional organizations and, 16–22
History of the Negro Race in America (Williams, 1882), 3
Homer G. Phillips Hospital (Missouri), 67
Hope, Justin, 7
Houston, E., 171
Howard, James Thomas, 97
Howard University (Washington, D. C.)
  influential figures in black psychiatry and, 6, 7, 8, 12, 201
  percentage of black psychiatrists in faculty of, 118
  percentage of black psychiatrists trained by, 110, 118
Hudson, George, 97

Indiana University School of Medicine, 14
Inner City Families: Development of Ego Under Stress (Lawrence, 1975), 129
Inpatient services, and department of psychiatry at Harlem Hospital, 31–34
Intelligence quotient testing, and racism, 89–90

James, Quinton, 131
James Comer Minority Research Fellowship, 139
Jenkins, Rose, 12, 130
Jenkins, Sidney, 15
JFK Center for Developmental Disabilities, 137
Johnson, Simon O., 4, 5, 9, 16
Johnson, Viola, 197
Joint Commission on Accreditation of Health Organizations (JCAHO), 186, 194–195
Joint Commission on Mental Health and Illness, 48
Jones, Billy, 11, 14, 20

Jones, James, 12
Jordan, Harold W., 11, 12
Justice, Ledro R., 97, 98

Karpman, Benjamin, 6–7
Keller, Jean, 35
Kennedy, Evelyn, 73
Kennedy, John F., 184–185
Kenney, Howard, 192
Kenney, John A., 4
Keyes, Gloria, 12, 13
King, Martin Luther, Jr., 104, 197
Koch, Ed, 59
Kolb, Lawrence, 26
Korean War, and black military psychiatrists, 96

Lakin State Hospital (West Virginia), 5, 9–10
Landy, Rosalie, 41
Law, and forensic psychiatry, 155
Lawrence, Leonard E., 14, 16, 22, 97, 98, 131
Lawrence, Margaret Morgan, 13, 31, 40, 129–130, 165
Lawson, William B., 20
Leal, Carol, 43, 131
Lewis, George Milton, 97
Lewis-Hall, Freda, 18
Lightfoot, Orlando, 170
Lincoln, Abraham, 96, 200
Lyons Veterans Administration Medical Center (New Jersey), 191

MacDonald, Lonnie, 28, 31, 35
Mackey, Elvin, 19, 20
Mallory, George, 12, 13, 17
Managed care, and mental health care for Black Americans, 208–210
Marks, Shirley, 16
Marshall University School of Medicine (West Virginia), 185–186
Martin Luther King Jr. Hospital, 12–13
Mashikian, Hagop S., 28, 31
Massachusetts State Advisory Committee for Mental Health and Retardation, 137

Index

Massenburg, Jerome, 97
Mattox, Gail, 13
Maultsby, Maxie C., Jr., 12
Maurice Falk Medical Foundation, 15
Mays, William R., 97
McKinney, Leon, 130
McMillan, Mae, 14, 129, 130
Medical Committee for Human Rights, 15
Medical schools. *See also* Academia; Education; Faculty; Teaching
  black psychiatrists as faculty, 114–116, 118–120
  black psychiatrists trained at foreign, 118
  development of department of psychiatry, 67–75
  percentage of faculty positions held by minorities, 141, 211
  recruitment of black students by, 110–113
Medicare, race and quality of hospital care, 91
Meharry Medical College
  black psychiatrists on faculty of, 118
  development of department of psychiatry
    atmosphere of, 70–71
    challenges facing department chairperson, 70
    curriculum of, 71–73
    decision making and, 71
    establishment of, 67–68, 75
    faculty of, 73–74
    recruited chair of, 12, 69, 75
    research and, 74
  percentage of black psychiatrists trained by, 110, 118
Menninger, Karl, 186, 188
Menninger, Will, 186
Mental health
  civil rights movement and studies of impact of racism on black Americans and, 15
  current issues affecting black Americans
    affirmative action and, 214
    health care reform and, 205–207
    managed care and, 208–210
  psychiatric research and, 211–212
  psychiatry as a career and, 207–208
  public policy in New York City, 59–62
  research on black populations and, 15, 78–79, 80–87, 142, 211–212
  training of staff at Harlem Rehabilitation Center and, 53–55
Mental Health Systems Act, 64
Mentors. *See also* Role models
  black psychiatrists in academia and, 211
  black research psychiatrists and, 144, 145, 211
Methodist Church, 67
Methodology, of survey on black psychiatrists in academia, 116–117
Michigan Center for Forensic Psychiatry, 155
Michigan State University, 13, 196
Miles, Carlotta, 131
Military psychiatry, and black psychiatrists
  Civil War and, 95–96
  combat stress behaviors and, 99–103
  duties of, 97–99
  experience of being black in military and, 103–104
  research on, 96–97
  in World War I to Vietnam era, 96
Military services, desegregation of, 8
Minnesota Multiphasic Personal Inventory (MMPI), and diagnosis of black patients, 82–83
Minority Group Program (American Psychiatric Association), 19, 20
Mitchell, Nellie, 131
Mitchell-Bateman, Mildred, 9–10, 13–14, 17, 21, 179–186
Moore, Austin, 39, 43
Morehouse School of Medicine (Georgia), 12, 13, 118
Moton, Robert R., 4

National Guard, 96
National Institute of Drug Abuse, 64
National Institute of Mental Health (NIMH)
  Center for Minority Group Mental Health Programs, 20

community psychiatry and, 49
Cuban/Haitian Mental Health Unit and American Psychiatric Association, 18
Harlem Rehabilitation Center and, 50
program to recruit minority medical students into psychiatry, 113–114
report on racism in 1973, 78
Veterans Administration's representative to Committee on Mental Health, 200
National Institutes of Health, 91, 144
National Joint Commission on Mental Health, 27
National Medical Association, 3, 15, 16, 134
New York City, and mental health services, 57–59, 62–63
New York State Office of Alcoholism Services, 62
Nickens, Herbert, 11–12
Norris, Donna M., 18, 132, 134, 135–136, 137–138, 171
Northampton Veterans Administration Medical Center (Massachusetts), 192–193
Nursing staff, and department of psychiatry at Harlem Hospital, 32, 38

Obstetrics and gynecology, and department of psychiatry at Harlem Hospital, 38–49
Onque, Gloria, 14
Operation Desert Storm, and military psychiatry, 102–103
Osteopathy, and Veterans Administration, 192, 196–197
Outpatient services, and development of department of psychiatry in general hospital, 29–31
Overholser, Winfred, 8
Oxley, Leo, 96

Paraprofessionals, training of mental health, 38, 53–55
Parker, Averette, 131
Parks, Gilbert, 18
Peal, James, 11

Peer Review Manual and *Peer Review Prelude and Promise* (American Psychiatric Association), 19
Perry, Richard, 41
Personal reminiscences, of black psychiatrists
on career in Veterans Administration, 187–202
of head of university department of psychiatry, 185–186
of state commissioner of mental health, 179–185
Phillips, George McKenzie, 11
Phillips, Robert T. M., 16, 19, 114
Physicians, percentage of black in U.S., 173
Pierce, Chester, 13, 17, 20, 21, 131
Pincus, Harold Alan, 19, 148
Pinder, Frank E., 13
Pinderhughes, Charles A., 3, 13, 14, 17, 18, 21, 170–171
Posttraumatic stress disorder (PTSD), 99, 101
Poussaint, Alvin, 13, 14, 15, 111
Powell, Gloria Johnson, 13, 74, 130
Powell, William, Jr., 96
Practice, black child psychiatrists and patterns of, 136–138. *See also* Clinical practice
Pregnancy, and Harlem Hospital program for unwed teenagers, 38–39
Prisons
percentage of blacks in population of, 153
work environments of forensic psychiatrists and, 155–158
Proctor, Charles, 74
Professional organizations. *See also* American Psychiatric Association
child and adolescent psychiatry and, 136–138
history of black leadership and, 16–22
psychoanalysis and, 171–172
representation of black psychiatrists in leadership of, 212–214
teaching opportunities for forensic psychiatrists and, 158

Program for Minority Research Training in Psychiatry (PMRTP), 19, 148–149
Prudhomme, Charles, 5, 7–9, 17, 21
Psychiatric Aspects of School Desegregation (Committee on Social Issues, 1957), 21
Psychiatric residency training, at Harlem Hospital, 36–37
Psychiatry. *See also* Black psychiatrists; Child and adolescent psychiatry; Community psychiatry; Department of psychiatry; Forensic psychiatry; Military psychiatry
  Black Americans and choice of as career, 207–208
  place of psychoanalysis in black, 163–165
  recruitment of black medical students into, 113–114
Psychoanalysis, and black psychiatrists
  future trends in, 173–174
  professional organizations and, 171–172
  publications and, 170–171
  role of in black psychiatry, 163–165
  survey of, 165–169, 172–173
  workplaces and, 169–170
Psychologists, training of at Harlem Hospital, 38
Psychopharmacology, and psychiatric education, 72
Public policy
  diversity in health care and, 91
  mental health issues in New York City and, 59–62
Public relations, and Veterans Administration, 195–196
Purvis, Charles, 96

Questionnaires, and surveys of black psychiatrists, 117–118, 165–166

Race, and anthropological use of term "ethnicity," 84
Racial discrimination. *See* Racism
Racism
  in academia, 126, 127
  child and adolescent psychiatry and, 134–135
  civil rights movement and studies of impact on mental health of black Americans, 15
  forensic psychiatry and, 156–158
  funding of black research psychiatrists and, 146
  military psychiatry and issues related to, 103–104
  National Institute of Mental Health report on in 1973, 78
  observations of psychiatrist from Africa on mental health issues in U.S. and, 87–91
  psychoanalysts and, 170–171
  research and training of black psychiatrists and, 145–146
  studies of mental health in black Americans and, 15, 78–79, 142
  Veterans Administration and black psychiatrists, 188–189
Racism and Mental Health (Willie, Kramer, and Brown, 1973), 8, 15
Rainbow-Earhart, Kathryn, 9, 10
Ralph, James, 14, 20
Randall, Jay, 96
Ransom, Raymond, 43
Rapier, John, 96
Raskin, Raymond, 36
Recreation groups, at Harlem Hospital, 41
Rehabilitation, and department of psychiatry at Harlem Hospital, 34–35. *See also* Harlem Rehabilitation Center
Research
  black psychiatrists in academia and, 121, 210–212
  department of psychiatry at Meharry Medical College and, 74
  on mental health issues in black community, 15, 78–79, 80–87, 142, 211–212
  survey of black psychiatrists as researchers, 141–149
Retirement, and career in Veterans Administration, 201–202
Review procedures, of department of psychiatry at Harlem Hospital, 39
Rickman, Edward, 12
Roberts, Esther, 11, 43

Robinson, Luther D., 9, 10, 12
Rockefeller, John D., 185
Role models, for black psychiatrists. *See also* Mentors
  in academia and research, 211
  education in child psychiatry and, 134
Rolfe, Daniel, 69
Rosenberger, John, 43
Ross, Phyllis Harrison, 14
Russell, Maurice V., 35

Sabshin, Melvin, 19
St. Elizabeth's Hospital (Washington, D. C.), 10
St. John's Mercy Medical Center (Missouri), 138
St. Louis University College of Medicine, 138
Sarpe, Betty, 73
Satisfaction, of black psychiatrists with academic careers, 120–123
Schizophrenia, research on overdiagnosis of in blacks, 81–82, 85
Schween, Audrey, 32
Sesame Street (television program), 131
Sexism. *See also* Women
  in academia, 126, 127
  state commissions of mental health and, 183–184
Sharpley, Robert, 113
Sheeley, Enid, 97
Sheps, Jack, 43, 44
Shervington, Walter, 11, 16
Silcott, William, 73
Simmons, Dorothea, 9, 131
Slaughter, Isaac, 20
Smith, Alan Percival, 5
Smith, Anna, 12
Smith, James Almer, III, 97, 98
Smith, Quentin Ted, 13, 131
Social services, and department of psychiatry at Harlem Hospital, 35
Social workers, training of, 37–38
Sociopsychiatric rehabilitation, philosophy of, 50–51
Solomon Carter Fuller Fellowship, 113
Solomon Carter Fuller, M.D. Award, 19
South Africa, and apartheid, 17–18
Spalding, Vernon, 95

Spurlock, Jeanne, 12, 14, 16, 17, 18, 19, 21, 22, 113, 129, 148, 169, 171
States, departments of mental health
  early appointments of black psychiatrists to administrative positions, 11
  personal reminiscences of commissioner in West Virginia, 179–185
Stevens, Rutherford, 21
Stewart, Altha, 20
Stewart, Gaston, 97
Substance abuse
  Harlem Hospital and inpatient treatment for pregnant women, 31
  Harlem Rehabilitation Center and, 52
  military psychiatry and, 100–102
  Veterans Administration and, 192, 196
Surveys, of black psychiatrists
  in academic positions, 116–127
  in child and adolescent psychiatry, 129–139
  in forensic psychiatry, 153–159
  psychoanalysis and, 163–174
  research and, 141–149

Taft State Hospital (Oklahoma), 9
Teaching, and forensic psychiatry, 158. *See also* Academia; Education; Faculty; Medical schools
Tenure, and black psychiatrists in academia, 119, 121–122
Thomas, Claudewell, 13
Thomas, Fern J., 97
Tilden, Toussaint, 4, 5
Togus Veterans Administration Hospital (Maine), 189–190
Tomes, Henry, 73
Toney, Ellis, 12, 13
Topeka Veterans Administration Medical Center (Kansas), 188–189
Training. *See* Education
Training in Psychiatry—Harlem Hospital Center (1965), 36–37
Transference, and black students of psychoanalysis, 167–168
Transitional neuropsychiatric treatment (TNT), and Veterans Administration, 190
Treatment, black child psychiatrists and patterns of, 135–136

Truman, Harry S., 8
Trussell, Ray E., 25–26
Tucker, Alpheus, 96
Tuerek, Isadore, 10–11
Turkey, schizophrenia in, 81–82
Turner, Guthrie, 95
Tuskegee Institute, 3
Tuskegee Veterans Administration Hospital (Alabama), 4, 7–8, 191
Tweed, Andre, 13

United Nation's Draft Program for a Decade of Action to Combat Racism and Racial Discrimination, 17
Universities. *See* Academia; Education; specific institutions
University of Colorado Health Sciences Center, 137
University of Massachusetts, 192
University of Michigan, 196
University of South Carolina School of Medicine, 138

Vallis, Alberta, 131
Verdell, Barbara, 33
Veterans Administration, personal reminiscences of career of black psychiatrist in, 187–202. *See also* Tuskegee Veterans Administration Hospital; specific locations
Veterans Affairs Medical Center, study of racial disparities in health care services, 91. *See also* specific locations
Vietnam War
  military psychiatry and, 96, 100–102
  Veterans Administration and psychiatric care, 201
Violence, perceptions of blacks and, 90–91
Volunteers in Service to America (VISTA), 181

Wagner, Robert F., 25
Walden, Robert, 10, 14
Walden University, 67
Walker, Benjamin, 97
Wall, Audrey, 74
Walter Reed Army Hospital, 96–97
Ward, Joseph H., 4
Washington, Booker T., 3
Weinberg, Jack, 18
Welsing, Frances Cress, 15, 131
Westborough State Hospital (Massachusetts), 3, 4
West Virginia, personal reminiscences of commissioner of mental health, 179–185
West Virginia University School of Medicine, 185
Whatley, David, 197
White, Jocelyn, 13
Whiting Forensic Institute (Connecticut), 154–155
Wilderson, Ernest, 41
Wilking, Virginia N., 31, 37
Wilkinson, Charles, 13, 14, 17, 20, 21
Williams, Daniel Hale, 3
Williams, Donald, 13
Williams, Ernest Y., 6–7, 12
Williams, Shirley, 7
Wilson, Roy, 11
Womack, William, 14, 18, 22
Women. *See also* Sexism
  as black psychiatrists in academia, 125–126, 143
  military psychiatry and issues specific to, 102–103
World War I and World War II, and black military psychiatrists, 96
Worrell, Audrey, 11
Wright, Harry H., 22, 132, 134, 138
Wymes, Michael, 97, 98

Yale University School of Medicine, 111
Younge, Eugene, Jr., 9, 16

Zeller, Charles A., 179
Zimberg, Sheldon, 42, 43
Zimmerman, Veva, 14

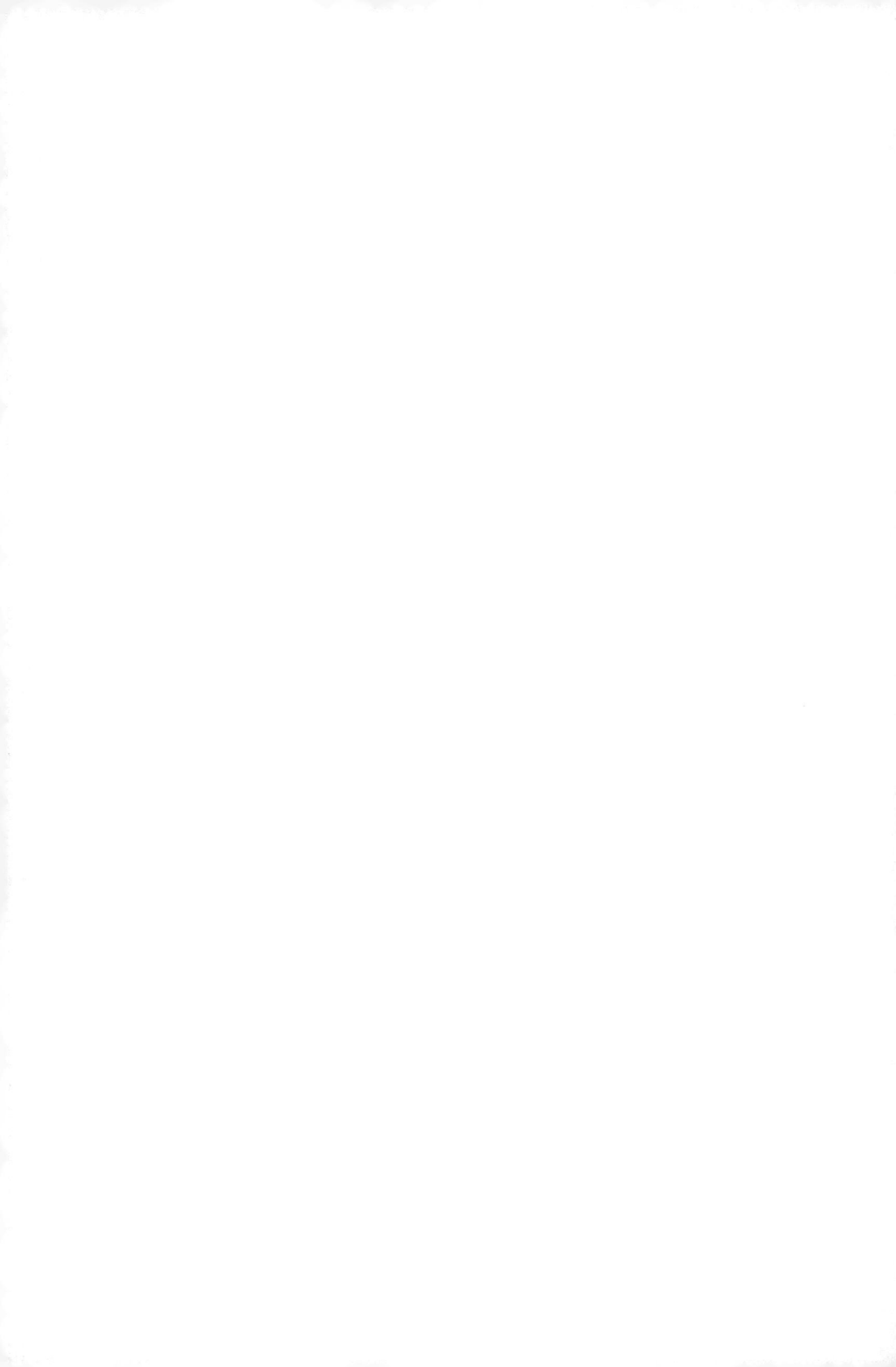

www.ingramcontent.com/pod-product-compliance
Ingram Content Group UK Ltd.
Pitfield, Milton Keynes, MK11 3LW, UK
UKHW021833210426
5322IPUK00011B/197/J